Functional Electromyography

Loren M. Fishman · Allen N. Wilkins

Functional Electromyography

Provocative Maneuvers in Electrodiagnosis

Springer

Loren M. Fishman, MD
College of Physicians & Surgeons
Columbia University
New York, NY 10028, USA
loren@sciatica.org

Allen N. Wilkins, MD
Manhattan Physical Medicine
and Rehabilitation
New York, NY 10013, USA

ISBN 978-1-4899-9141-6 ISBN 978-1-60761-020-5 (eBook)
DOI 10.1007/978-1-60761-020-5
Springer New York Dordrecht Heidelberg London

Printed on acid-free paper

Springer is part of Springer Science+Business Media (www.springer.com)

To our steadfast families

All that is constant is change.
– Ancient Chinese proverb

Love is not love that alters where it alteration finds.
– William Shakespeare

This book provides operational definitions for three commonly encountered medical conditions that currently lack precise criteria. It accomplishes this task by introducing common sense methods for measuring positional changes in electrophysiological metrics.

The authors make an effort to convince the reader of the practical, theoretical and historical fittingness of these further extensions of the physical examination, through anatomical analysis and empirical means, using imaging techniques and series of patients diagnosed and treated according to the methods proposed here.

The book's third and final aim is to suggest guidelines for the electromyographer who wishes to apply these new techniques to novel, and perhaps less frequently seen situations in clinical medicine.

Acknowledgment

The authors wish to thank Donell Hutson for his deft and decidedly patient treatment of the illustrations, the clear and steady guidance of Richard Lansing, our editor at Springer, Diana Schneider for putting all of us together, our colleagues for their many helpful comments, and our families for everything else.

Preface

In the course of electrodiagnostic examinations over what is, taken together, more than 30 years of practice, we have noticed changes in what were ostensibly immutable parameters. An individual's nerve conduction velocities or occasionally absolute or interpeak latencies in somatosensory-evoked potentials seemed at times to vary with position. Over the past 10 years, we have tried to study these inconstancies and to link these changes with their probable cause. In this book we present three of them very much the way we encountered them: in the course of clinical work, as extensions of the physical examination.

Our coming across these phenomena is, in a small way, parallel to what has happened in electromyography, and what may happen in science in general. Periods of confusion and disorder were followed by consolidation, standardization, and the drive to achieve a consensus in conceptual approach as well as methods and results. An unorganized, chaotic era of independent inquiry leads, inexorably, toward a unified theory, much as a cooling planet is thrown off to circle a molten sun. Then the subject, in our case electrodiagnosis, like a new planet, gets solid, as it were, and soon able to support practical activity, much as a stable world enables animated processes such as life itself. And following this, in the science as well as a new world, a second era of disorganized, exploratory activity begins.

In this book, we have taken advantage of the broadly accepted and largely stable metrics and parameters of electrodiagnosis in order to present a reasonably novel measure of a type of neuropathology. We have used a method based on unchanging techniques to record and interpret exactly the opposite: to document changes. We hope that if these observations are borne out by future work, then the methods described here will eventually join the expanding body of reliable tools of the clinical electromyographer.

Contents

Chapter 1
Electricity in Medicine: Philosophy Meets Physiology

> *The history of electrodiagnosis and electromyography has been one of increasing quantification on diminishing areas; from the millisecond impulse of the faradic coil to the hundredth millisecond impulse of the electronic generator; from the large percutaneous electrode to the barely visible tip of a needle; from the muscle to the muscle fiber. It would seem that we have reached the limits of minuteness in time and tip. But the one great lesson of the history of science is that the boundaries of knowledge are not fixed [1].*

Abstract Electricity was used therapeutically long before it took on a diagnostic role. Historically, electrodiagnosis began after the twin births of neurophysiology and the physics of electricity itself in the late eighteenth century. Their early developments were closely related, the first battery being designed after the electric fish, and early theories of motility imagining muscles much like condensers. When each subject evolved to independent and reliable principles, then one (electrical measurement) could be used to study the other (neurophysiology) and electrodiagnosis began. This chapter relates the confused but determined efforts of brilliant and above all determined individuals, at times generating more heat than light, but always seeking to understand our subject.

Keywords Electrodiagnosis · Neurophysiology · Luigi Galvani · Alessandro Volta · Julius Bernstein · Electron · Action potential · Injury current · Differential rheotome · Torpedo · Voltaic cell · Leyden jar · Animal electricity · Carlo Matteucci · Resting potential · Variably permeable membrane · ISEK · EMG

The history of electrophysiology, like a good deal of history, is peppered with false starts and stops, lulls due to factors scientific, temporal, political, and other, accidental happenstance that led to explosive insight. It also illustrates the inseparable relationship between technological advancement and scientific discovery.

This history reveals the place of electrodiagnosis in the neurological examination. It also shows that scientific inquiry both followed the linear progression of improved technology, and leapt discontinuously from new insights to underlying principles.

L.M. Fishman, A.N. Wilkins, *Functional Electromyography*,
DOI 10.1007/978-1-60761-020-5_1, © Springer Science+Business Media, LLC 2011

The groping turns that our understanding has taken may remind us that what seems factual today may appear fatuous tomorrow. Although our reasoning may *seem* linear to us, based as it is on accepted principles set forth from those who came before, progress is only possible if we are open to other possibilities and explanations.

Electricity and Medicine Grew Up Together

Electricity Through History: Minerals

Neanderthals

The recognition that there was something special about electricity and magnetism probably antedates recorded history. Amber, a fossilized resin from certain coniferous trees, which coated the Baltic Basin 6 or 7 million years ago [2], attracts light objects if given an electrostatic charge by vigorous rubbing. Neanderthals (ca. 600,000–350,000 BCE) are believed to have known this, since amber had a prominent place in their religious ornamentation.

Ancients: Sacred and Electrostatic

Lightning strikes down dissenters in virtually all mythologies, its power generally reserved for the gods. Evidence of humans' naïve acquaintance with these phenomena begins ca. 9,000 BC, when the attractive (electrostatic or magnetic) properties of minerals such as amber, lodestone, and magnetite were indicated.

This attractive property is also evidenced in its Arabic and Persian names, karabé and karubé, respectively, words meaning literally "to pull straw [3]." It also attracted attention from poets and sages. Thales of Miletus, the pre-socratic often credited with discovering that a diameter bisects a circle, remarked in 600 BC that, "elektron is endowed with a soul which draws light bodies until itself like a breath, and is nourished by them [3]." The word "electric" derives from the Greek word for amber: "ηλεκτρον" (elektron), and the mineral was used topically (generally in the form of jewelry) to treat headaches, arthralgia, and other bodily disorders [3].

The Bible

Genesis and *Numbers* refer to "electric force." In the story of the ark, very specific instructions are given for its construction, detailing the wooden tabernacle encrusted with and topped by continuous overlays of a conducting metal: gold. During storms at sea, unauthorized persons were prohibited from touching the arc, as the fire that surrounded it would cause certain death to those who touched this veritable lightening rod. The only persons authorized to enter the tabernacle during these times were the Levite priests who could somehow withstand its powers. It is illustrative to view the description of the arc's construction alongside the proscribed priestly garb, including an impressive suit of gold trailing to the floor, in effect grounding them, and since electrons are mutually repellent, insulating them from electrical demise [3].

Electrophysiology Through History: Animals

The Electric Fish

Beyond simple minerals and atmospheric events, those in ancient times were acquainted with the force of electricity generated by certain sea creatures. These creatures (certain eels, rays, and other fish) were collectively dubbed *narke* or "numbness-producers" by the Greeks, *torpedo* or "to render sluggish or inert" by Latin speakers, and *arimna* or "something that deprives of motion" by South American Indians [3]. These denizens of the deep produced shocks powerful enough to immobilize large mammals. The "technology" at this point was crude: the application of one animal (the live black torpedo) to another (a human) was used to stimulate muscles and numb the limbs [4]. Not aware of electricity per se, the ancients saw and felt muscular contraction after contact with the live torpedoes, and the fleeting sensory deficit.

The Roman physician Scribonus Largus (AD 46) used these electric fish to treat gout and headaches. Application of this technology was still fairly basic, as the numbing technique required the presence of a disagreeable, live marine animal [4]. A prescription from Scribonus may have read as follows:

> For any type of gout a live black torpedo should, when the pain begins, be placed under the feet. The patient must stand on a moist shore washed by the sea [*note precautions to keep the torpedo alive*] and he should stay like this until his whole foot and leg up to the knee is numb. This takes away present pain and prevents pain from coming on if it has not already arisen. In this way Anteros, a freedman of Tiberius, was cured [3].

Electric animal treatments continued well into the seventeenth century and broadened in their application. Various physicians turned to the electric fish for cephalgias and arthralgias, eplilepsy, vertigo, migraine, melancholy, and even prolapsus ani [3]. Indian physicians used the fish to treat "excess heat" [4] (Fig. 1.1).

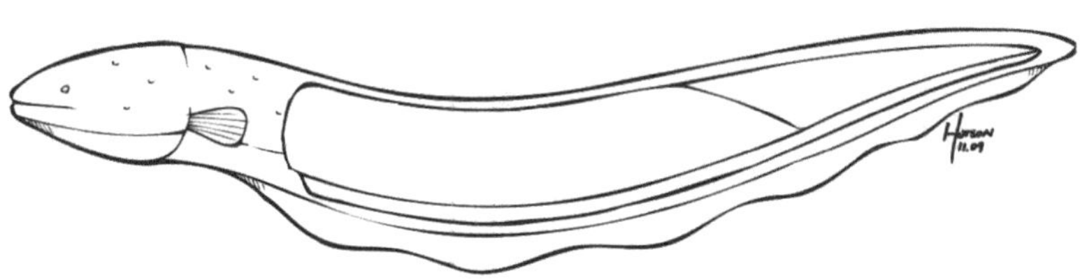

Fig. 1.1 The torpedo or electric fish

This fish inspired some physicians, and writers, and philosophers as well. Pliny, in his *Natural History*, marveled that

> [The torpedo] knows its own force and power, and being itself not benumbed, is able to astonish others .... From a considerable distance even, and if only touched with a spear or a staff this fish has the power of benumbing even the most vigorous arm, and of riveting the feet of a runner, however swift he may be in the race [3].

While the poet Oppian recited in the Haliutca that

The Cramp-Fish, when the pengent pain alarms,
Exerts his magick Pow'rs and poison'd Charms,
Clings around the Line, and bids th' Embrace infuse
From fertile Cells compress his subtil Juice
Th' aspiring Tide its restless Volume rears,
Rols up the steep Ascent of slipp'ry Hairs
Then fwn the Rod with easy Motion slides
And entering in the Fisher's Hand subsides.
On every joint and icy siffness steals,
The flowing Spirits inds, and Blood congeals
Down drops the Rod dismist, and floating lies,
Drawn captive in its Turn, the Fish's Prize [3].

Evidence of Electricity Through History: Beginning to Understand

Fascinating and useful though it was, this curative force was not given a name until 1600. In this year, William Gilbert of Colchester (physician to Queen Elizabeth I) used the term *electrica* to describe the excitation of amber in his publication, *De Magnete*, and to describe any substances that had properties reminiscent of amber. He also distinguished between electric and magnetic forces [3].

Half a century later, scientists inquired about how the sea animals were actually generating this observed electric force. In 1666, Francesco Redi observed that the shock delivered by an electric ray appeared to originate from two particular sickle-shaped muscles. Redi also established that though electricity *is* generated from muscles, maggots *do not* spontaneously generate from rotting meat [2] (Fig. 1.2).

Instrumental in the increasingly popular electrical research was the ability to isolate electricity into the lab, without live marine animals on the scene. Before the

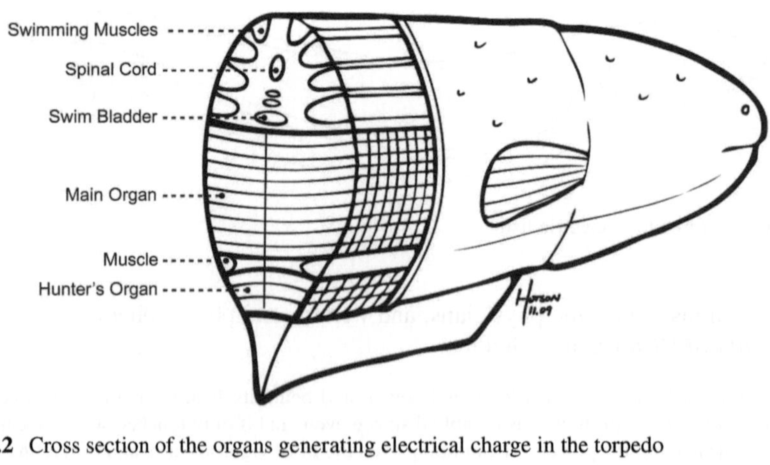

Fig. 1.2 Cross section of the organs generating electrical charge in the torpedo

mid-1700s, the best man-made approximations of electricity were crude electrostatic induction machines pioneered by Gilbert and Otto von Guericke. Guericke, for example, rotated a sulfur-filled globe against his hand to generate static electricity [3].

The practical use of electricity probably began in 1745 in Leyden with Pieter van Musschenbroek using a partially water-filled container topped by a cork with a nail protrusion to store electrical charge. Georg von Kleist of Cammin also supported the Leyden jar [3], which gave the scientific community a portable, readily available quantity of electricity, in essence by adding a capacitor to the existing electrostatic generators [4], moving electrical study away from the ocean and into labs.

That same year, a 21-year-old student named Kratzenstein heard his professor, J.C. Krueger suggest that electricity might treat paralysis. Kratzenstein applied static electricity to a woman with a chronically contracted finger, successfully relieving the contraction and enabling her to play the harpsichord once again [2]. Some, forgetting the torpedo, assert him to be the first person to use electricity therapeutically [4]. The king of Denmark later forced him into a career of electrotherapy, despite his primary interest in basic sciences [1]. He published the first report of individually stimulated muscle contraction with static electricity in 1745. The noted powers of electricity had swung like a pendulum from paralyzing muscles to activating them.

Now equipped with portable electric generators, physicians began using electricity as an analgesic, and to treat paralysis, hemiplegia, kidney stones, sciatica, and angina pectoris, to name a few [4]. Schrechter remarked that "electricity was extolled for just about any flagging bodily viscus or aperture." [2] Nollett advised that it could be used to "chase from the body the vicious humors causing all sicknesses." [2]

As doctors and scientists were busy with the therapeutic uses of electricity, physiologists probed muscular function with it. As we will examine later in this book, introducing a technique as treatment may precede diagnostic use.

Quickly becoming the hottest topic in medicine, electricity was tried as a cure for almost any medical ailment conceivable. Over 25 papers on electricity in medicine were seen between 1750 and 1780 in the *Journal de Medicine* alone [4].

Electricity was considered vaguely magical at this time; possibly able to reanimate the dead. When 3-year-old Catherine Sophia Greenhill was pronounced dead after a fall from her first story window in 1774:

> With the consent of the parents [Mr Squires] very humanely tried the effects of electricity. At least *twenty minutes* had elapsed before he could apply the shock, which he gave to various parts of the body without any apparent success; but at length, upon transmitting a few shocks through the thorax, he perceived a small pulsation: soon after the child began to sigh, and to breathe, though with great difficulty. In about ten minutes she vomited: a kind of stupor, occaisioned by the depression of the cranium, remained for some days, but proper means being used, the child was restored to perfect health and spirits in about a week.
>
> Mr. Squires gave this astonishing case of recovery to the above gentlemen, from no other motive than a desire of promoting the good of mankind; and hopes for the future that no person will be given up *for dead*, till various means have been used for their recovery. The girl probably sustained a head injury. the electricity may have awakened her from deep coma rather cardiac defibrillation [5].

The convent battery prompted further attempts at reanimation, usually of recently executed criminals. Giovani Aldini of London, nephew of the famous Galvani (whom we will meet shortly) was a leader in these controversial experiments. The idea of electric revival spread beyond the medical community and into the culture, inspiring Mary Shelley in her creation of *Frankenstein* [6].

Animal Electricity Controversy

In the scientific community, the questionable benefits of reanimating executed criminals paled before the real controversy about the concept of "animal electricity." Was electricity a force intrinsic to animals, a force that they generated, or simply a force to which animals were subject, as anything else? Animal electricity smacked of the obscure, pre-scholastic notion of an inaccessible and unknowable entity akin to the soul; empirically oriented group saw electricity as a force of physics, with no spiritual association at all. Yet biology is a science too.

Luigi **Galvani**, a tragic and influential figure in the history of science, intensively studied the relationship between electricity and muscle contraction in frogs, performing countless experiments [7]. He became interested in this phenomenon after incidentally observing, in 1786, that the muscle in his frog preparation contracted vigorously in response to a spark leaping from an electrical generator when his wife walked across his lab with a metallic knife in her hand (see Fig. 1.3 for details) [6].

Wanting to make sure the effect was indeed electric in nature, Galvani turned to the other known source of electricity at the time: atmospheric lightning

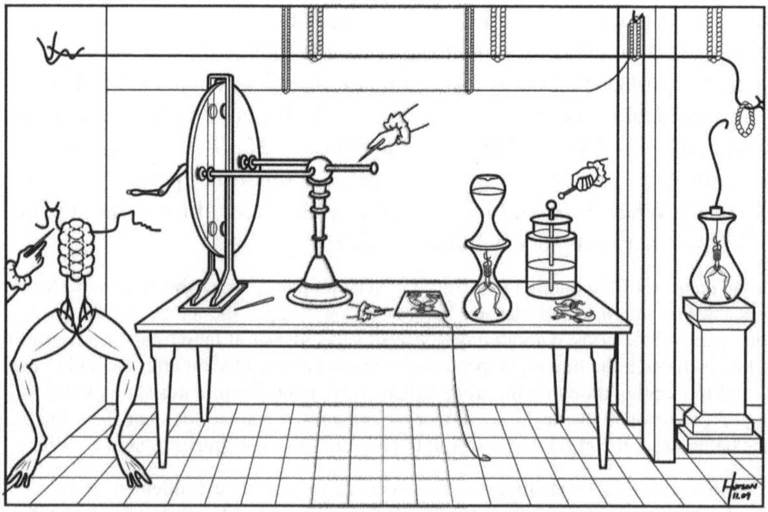

Fig. 1.3 A spark apparently leapt from the generator to the knife blade that Luigi Galvani's wife held to the exposed nerve of the frog. The spark somehow bridged the gap, releasing the electrical energy and causing the muscle to contract

demonstrated to be electric by Benjamin Franklin in 1750 [6]. Galvani succeeded in using such a meterological event to cause a frog's leg to twitch.

He believed that body-generated "animal electricity" explained how creatures move, but also that this was a natural and knowable force. The only object scientists of the time knew to be capable of holding electricity were Leyden jars, and to Galvani, the muscle had similar properties. In his model, the frog muscle stored electricity, functioning as the body's capacitor or "Leyden jar." The nerve's membrane divided the internal surface from the external one, creating a potential electrical disequilibrium.

In Galvani's mind, animal electricity derived from nervous tissue itself, particularly brain tissue, and was conducted along "oil-coated" nerves (to prevent dispersion) on its way to the Leyden jars of the body, the muscles. The nerves themselves were viewed as capacitors, considered too small to retain or generate enough electricity to power contractions of the magnitude observed in the frogs. His "frog current" was a muscle current, not attributed to the nerves themselves at all. Galvani believed that an external spark from his lab generator enabled the internal electricity to flow, inducing muscle contraction [7]. Exactly how muscles came to use their electricity was another, essentially unanswered question.

His theories initially met with much excitement and acceptance. When Alessandro **Volta** first read his commentaries in 1792, he gushed "it contains one of the most beautiful and surprising discoveries and the germ of many others." [1] Though initially skeptical, "he had changed from incredulity to fanaticism" after successfully repeating some of the experiments himself. By the following year, however, Volta, along with Bassiano Carminati, had their own disparate theories.

Volta and others (e.g., Monro and Fowler) postulated that the electricity observed was not "animal electricity" spontaneously generated by an animal's muscle, as Galvani suggested, but was instead generated by an artificial electric circuit set up by the two different metal plates in the experimental set-up and connected by animal tissue or water. This was electricity, but it never came from animals. Animals were simply passive conductors [6]. Volta promoted his point by connecting a bimetallic arc to two points on a nerve and causing contraction without contacting the muscle itself at all. He concluded that contractions did not require current flow from inside to outside of the muscle, as implied by Galvani's muscle-as-Leyden-jar theory [7].

Following Johannes Mueller's observations that stimulating different types of nerves produced different physiological effects, Volta further challenged the theory of muscle-and-nerve-as-capacitor through a sensory nerve on his own tongue. When Volta placed the bimetallic arc on his tongue, he experienced a sour taste for the duration of the metallic contact [7]. Were the tongue functioning as a capacitor, it should eventually exhaust its discharge, and thus the sour taste. The lasting flavor in this experiment seemed to disprove Galvani's theory.

Galvani was not convinced. In 1794 he demonstrated the direct generation of electricity in an animal tissue by placing the frog's leg in one container and the nerve in another, observing contraction with a variety of non-metallic connectors [7]. He showed contractions using a monometallic arc, a piece of tissue and even direct connection of nerve to muscle surface [7]. Galvani's decisive experiment of 1797 in which he elicited frog contraction by connecting the sciatic nerves of two different frog legs, went tragically unnoticed [7] (see Fig. 1.4). In fact this seminal experiment also indicates, admittedly broadly, that comparable stimuli may activate different nerves, suggesting a number of contemporary concepts such as the universal nature of neurotransmission, and the synapse itself.

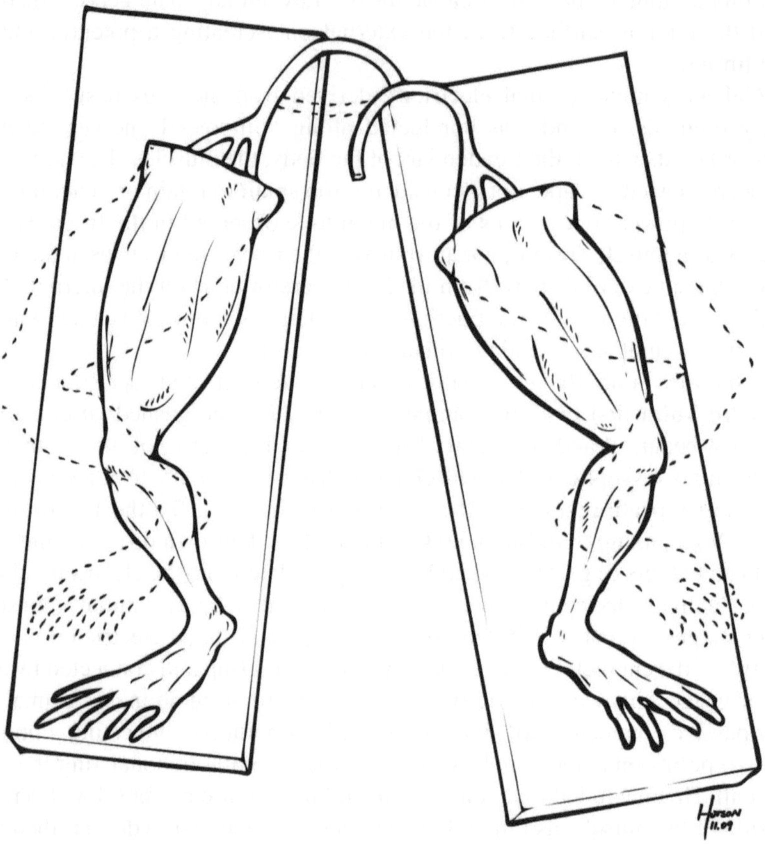

Fig. 1.4 Picture of two frogs' legs' sciatic nerves in contact. Luigi Galvani refuted the claim that all electricity came from metallic interaction by demonstrating that one sciatic nerve induced muscular contraction in another [7]

From our vantage point we may easily distinguish between Galvani's theory of nerve and muscle as capacitor and the general proposition that electricity is a physiological force generated within live organisms, which might have many different explanations. This oversight may be excused, considering that there was nearly total ignorance of both electricity and physiology! Galvani's and Volta's views could be reconciled by conceding that while animals were not the *sole* source of electricity, they were *a* source. The similarities between muscle tissue and the organs of electric fish were compelling. Galvani was touching on the idea that nerves can convey enough electricity to stimulate muscles to release their energy (see Fig. 1.4).

Well on his way to becoming an authority on the physics of electricity, Volta responded that dissimilar metals may be unnecessary, but humid, heterogeneous substances of some kind (present in each of the aforementioned experiments) were necessary and sufficient to produce the electricity required to induce muscle contraction [7].

1. Around this time, Volta was also working on electrical generation. Having vastly improved the electrometer and attempting to generate more electricity by stacking metal components between discs of moist paper, he invented the "pile," better known as a "battery," in 1799 [7].
2. This invention represented another milestone in electrical studies, as the device was capable of reliably generating electricity, exponentially improving empirical research on the subject. But instead of disproving Galvani's theories, Volta was actually giving an example of biophysics.

Ironically, it was the stack of modular components seen in the electric organ of the fish previously mentioned that inspired the construction of Volta's initial battery: metal parts separated by humid discs. Despite the influence of the fish on the creation of his battery, *Volta maintained that even the electricity observed from this fish was simply the "common" type of electricity, and not "animal" in any way* [7]. Because the fish organ and the battery operated by the same principles ("alternation of different conductors acting as motors of electricity"), Volta came to the conclusion that the action in the fish was not specific to animals [7],though he dubbed his own device, "artificial electric organ." [2] (see Fig. 1.2).

It would seem that to Volta, the connotation of "animal electricity," brought to mind the mysterious "unknowables" of the Middle Ages. One need only recall the ancient belief that lightning itself was hurled by a deity. Although Volta sought to demystify electricity, to understand it, Galvani was not his opposite. He did not see things in the Medieval way. Galvani must have believed in electricity as a physical force also to construct the lightning experiment, let alone interpret its results as he did. The difference between the men was that Volta sought to understand electricity, and Galvani was using electricity to understand something else: biology. Both men were objective empiricists. The tragedy is that Galvani was working from the opposite side, the biological side, with the same fundamental conviction: electrical phenomena, biological and otherwise, can be understood.

After its creation, the battery presented so many exciting possibilities that it both overshadowed Galvani's frog-current studies, and gave additional credibility to his opponent, Alessandro Volta. Volta was a modern man, writing in the French, English, and German journals of the day and speaking at large secular gatherings about electricity as physics. Galvani's non-conformity, his atheism, his poverty, may have led to his untimely death. Neither saw, as we might today, that the laws of physics were never broken, yet biological systems are explicable through electrochemistry.

In the Italy of the time the fierce controversy—supporters of Galvani and supporters of Volta—was fuelled—as perhaps such controversies often are—by a lack of imagination sufficient to render the views compatible. The two men differed in their views of the source of the electricity that caused muscular contractions, but actually each man used the others domain as an essential part of his work: Galvani looked at the frog's muscle as a biological equivalent of the Leyden jar, and Volta used the frog's leg as a galvanometer! The question was whether electrically stimulated muscle contraction represented a biological process or a mere application of physics to biological systems. Did electrical stimulation of muscle contraction mimic a natural process, or was it like painting a herring red, proving that paint worked on fish, but demonstrating nothing particular about the herring?

Before long, two stunningly accurate experiments delivered a temporary *coup de grace* to Galvani's theory: one measuring the speed of electrical conduction as comparable to the speed of light, the other delimiting the speed of nerve conduction. It seemed that what was called animal electricity could not be electricity at all, and the Galvanists retreated in confusion. Animal electricity studies were largely abandoned for the next three decades [7], lying in wait for better instruments of measure and Bernstein's theory of a variably permeable neuronal membrane to emerge.

Modern understanding of the complexities of electrical involvement in nerve and muscle physiology would have been difficult to confirm within the confines of eighteenth-century technology [8]. Though Galvani misplaced the source of animal electricity, he correctly based his life's work on the theory that electrical energy was generated within the body and relied on nerves for activation [8].

Technological Advances in Medicine

In the early nineteenth century, "electropuncture"—applying electricity through inserted needles—was developed and advanced by Sarlandiere and d'Etilles [4]. Magiendie similarly applied this technique at specific Japanese acupuncture points [2]. Electropuncture was used to treat fistulas, bleeding, and tumors [2], not unlike today's electrocautery. This methodology was valuable for research; needles were an excellent way to identify nerve and muscle impulses [2]. Guillaume Duchenne de Boulogne devoted his life to electrostimulation, and devised cloth covered electrodes to avoid painful needles [4]. Some of his kindness might have arisen because more than once he induced contractions strong enough to fracture cervical vertebrae [1].

Using these electrodes, Duchenne systematically mapped out the function of most of the facial muscles. Though his interest was in therapy, his hard work and creativity pioneered many of the early devices of electrodiagnosis [1].

Volta's "victory" over animal electricity slowed electrophysiology for many years, the means for producing and detecting electricity were also sluggish. The galvanometer, used to detect and measure small electric currents, was not invented until the 1820s, and was not practically useful until the 1830s [1]. Furthermore, the therapeutic uses of electricity of the early and mid nineteenth century seemed to be put on hold while the animal electricity controversy alternately slumbered and raged [4].

The invention of the galvanometer was critical in the forward motion of electrodiagnostics. In 1838, Carlo Matteucci used the improved device to demonstrate conclusively that when electrodes touched a cut surface and intact membrane of a contracting muscle, electricity was indeed generated [1, 6], validating some of Galvini's original claims on the existence of animal-generated electricity. He also showed that stimulating three frogs' muscles in series elicited three times the response, even if stimulus strength did not change [6]. This demonstration gave further credence to the idea that contraction was more than an artifact of electrode cell contact; there were three muscles with only two contact points, yet the current tripled. This was the turning point, when it became clear that electrical impulses excited a response in nerve or muscle intrinsic to the physiology of creatures. Electricity was not powering the response; rather, electricity was a stimulus, triggering a response (Fig. 1.5).

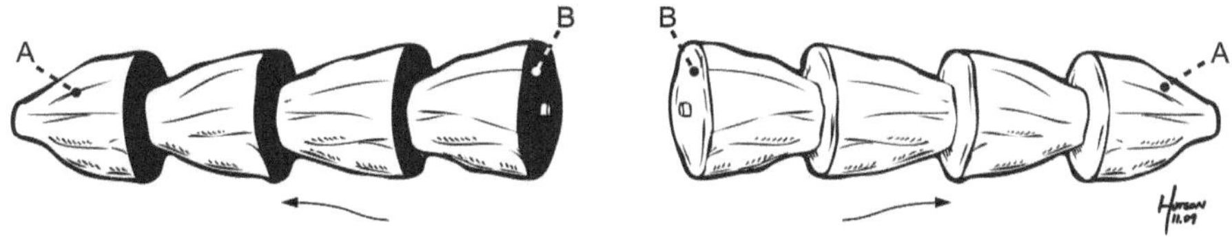

Fig. 1.5 By varying the number of muscles he linked in series between A and B, Matteucci elicited an electrical potential proportional to the muscle mass, not the stimulus, suggesting that "animal electricity" was the source

What was the underlying principle in this impressive experiment? Immaculate replication and careful measurement implied great attention to detail, it is true, but the heart of this demonstration was that Matteucci identified and varied the proper independent variable: how many muscles were aligned and found that the dependent variable—the amount of electricity generated—varied proportionately. Also of considerable significance are the metrics, such as conduction velocity, that did not change. Galvani neither had the technical resources to even approximate nerve conduction velocity nor the "all or nothing" principle or other parameters of nerve conduction and muscle response. These were critical to later investigators, to whom we shall now turn. But we shall meet this principle again later in the book.

Dubois-Reymond wound 5 km of wire over 24,000 turns to create a sensitive galvanometer, to measure the voltage potential in resting muscle. He described an "action current" that accompanies every contraction of muscle, possibly the earliest recording of the "action potential" [9]. A few years later in 1851, he performed what was essentially the first EMG. With liquid-filled jars as electrodes, he detected action currents from a contracting arm [1]. It was not until 1890, however, that Etienne made the first actual recording of this activity.

Despite the prevailing belief that the speed of impulses traveling along nerves—viewed as "simple" conductors of electricity—should be impossible to measure, as they are likely akin to light [6] and thus travel impossibly fast, German scientist Hermann von Helmholtz perhaps was not paying attention. In 1850 he successfully measured the time required for a nervous impulse to travel a short distance [6]. His device started the clock with a stimulus, stopped the clock with the twitch of a frog's leg at two different points. He then subtracted the differences in time and distance [6], much the way electromyographers measure today, and with comparable results! Direct nerve impulse measurement brought a biological metric previously "unreachable" by modern science to everyone's lab bench.

Learning the actual speed of propagation, however, opened questions about the nature of nerve conduction. The recorded speeds were far slower than the speed of light propagation or electrical fields [6]. If nerve conduction were electrical, why did it travel so slowly?

Du Bois-Reymond found nerve conduction similar to "injury currents"—the always negative currents that flowed from injured areas of tissue. He set about to measure the conduction velocity of this "negative variation." If conduction down a nerve were an advancing region of negative potential, one should be able to detect it. Unfortunately he was unsuccessful [10]. Possibly this was due to the slow, insensitive galvanometers available.

It took Julius Bernstein, a pupil of both von Helmholtz and du Bois-Reymond, and his differential rheotome to get a picture of nerve conduction. Bernstein developed a marvelously ingenious mechanical solution to compensate for the galvanometers' electrical failings. For the sheer cleverness of it, a few words of explanation are in order. His device had two sets of electrodes, one stimulating set of which were located at one spot on the nerve, and a second recording set located some distance away. The two recording electrodes each ended in a pin attached to an armature that was attached to a pulley, causing it to rotate. Each pin spent most of its time rotating and exposed to air, thus creating a broken circuit (resulting in no recording from the nerve). For a portion of its arc, each passed through a small mercury bath that occupied only a tiny portion of the circumference traversed by each spinning pin; the mercury served as a commutator, and closed the circuit when the respective pins crossed through the pool, breaking it again when the pin exited the mercury [10] (Figs. 1.6 and 1.7).

Stimulation of the nerve was by way of a similar pin arrangement on the other side of the armature; depending on the speed of rotation and the size of the mercury pool. The stimulation rate and duration could be adjusted. The temporal delay between stimulation and recording was adjusted not only by the speed of revolution but also by the angle between the two armature radii; the larger the angle, the longer the delay; if the angle were 180°, stimulation and recording occurred simultaneously. Looking at windows of time revealed when the wave front passed, enabling one to calculate conduction velocity down the nerve. This also facilitated measuring the duration of depolarization at each point by adjusting the recording windows. In order to overcome the problem of insensitivity of the galvanometer, Bernstein could spin the armature rapidly, thus stimulating multiple depolarizations in a short period

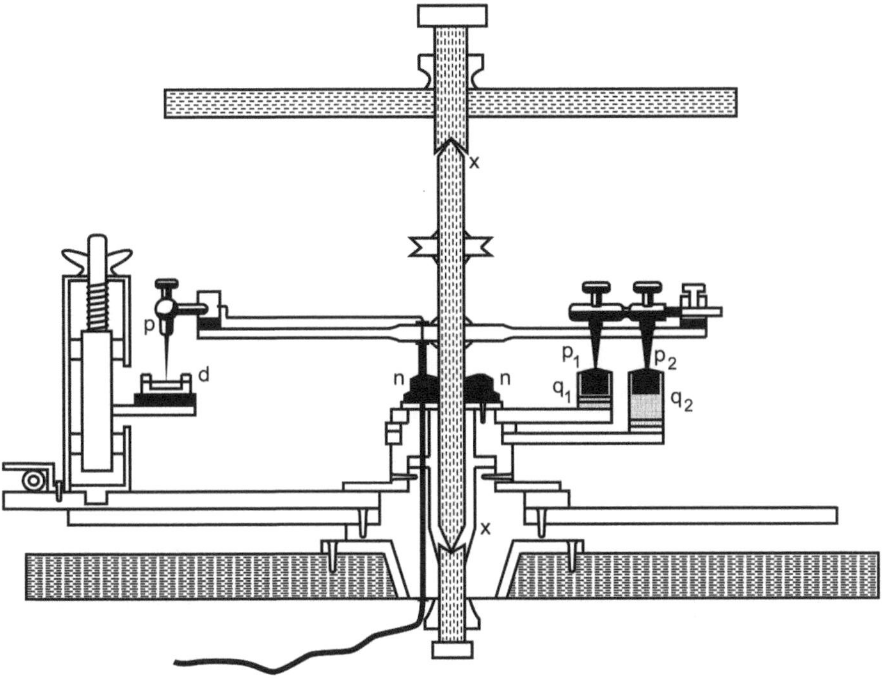

Fig. 1.6 Julius Bernstein's Rheotome: The pin p went through the mercury dish d to complete the stimulation circuit. Pins p_1 and p_2 completed the recording circuit as they moved through q_1 and q_2. Timing depended on the angle between the dishes, and the speed of rotation around the axis x–x

of time and accumulating enough of them to be recognized by the instrument, a sort of summation akin to averaging [10] (Fig. 1.8).

With this technique Bernstein demonstrated that the time of depolarization was about a millisecond, and that the propagation speed of depolarization equaled the speed of nerve conduction, strongly suggesting they were one and the same. The differential rheotome yielded estimated the speed of conduction and also the duration of depolarization [10].

From these experiments it appeared likely that nerve propagation was an electrical event, but the mechanism was not simple: nerve current did not seem to follow the known laws of electric current propagation [6]—it was much too slow.

There were many theories at the time attempting to explain this disparity. Ludimar Von Hermann (another student of Dubois-Reymond), for example, proposed the "local circuit theory," [6] based on the Galvani-like idea that the nerve fiber consisted of a conductive core separated from an external fluid phase by a relatively insulating coating, and that any electrical disturbance originating in a nerve could influence near regions through a local current loop involving the internal core,

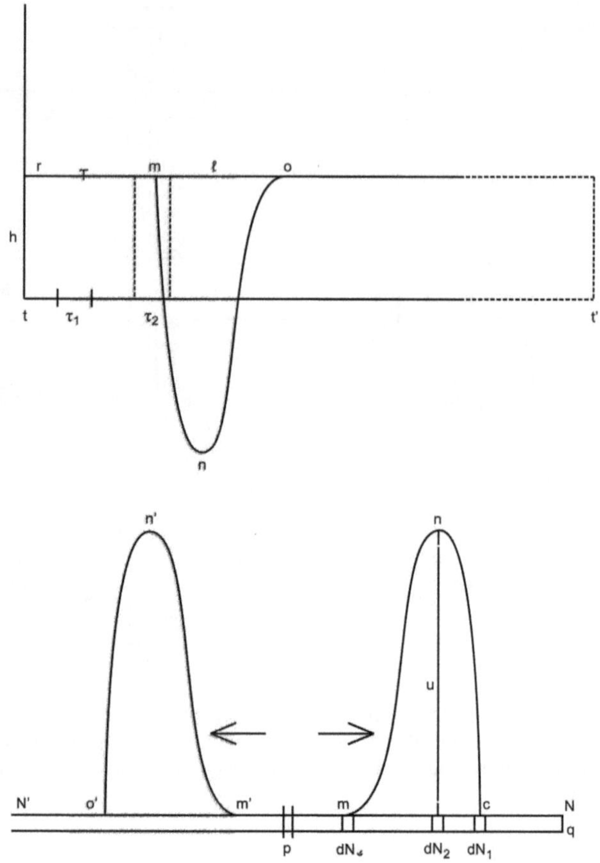

Fig. 1.7 Above: Bernstein's recording of the action current. *Below*: Plots representing the magnitude of the action current as a function of distance along the axon at a given time

the insulating sheet, and the external fluid [6]. Similar to the injury current running from the positive outside to the negative inside of a cell, if there were an area that depolarized—the area of "negative variation"—a current could run from the positive area outside the nerve to the negative area within, setting up local currents which in turn would induce the nerve's adjacent areas to depolarize (Fig. 1.9).

Walther Nernst showed that electrical potentials could be generated by differences in chemical concentration. Drawing on that, and another few decades of experience following his invaluable and ingenious work just cited, Bernstein postulated that excitable cells generate a transmembrane electrical potential by virtue of selective permeability and the differences in ionic concentration it creates. Excitation consists of the disappearance of this selective permeability, resulting in potassium moving out of the cell and sodium moving in, and a propagating impulse along the membrane [6] essentially what we believe today.

In a sense, Galvani's capacitor-theory has been changed into a long, thin, cylindrical, and variably resistant capacitor, with electrical negativity traveling

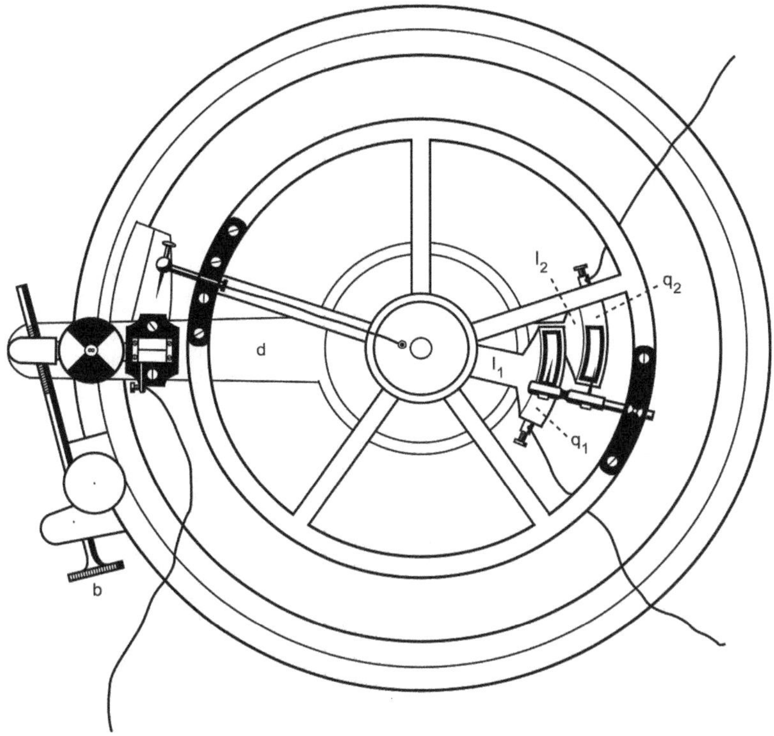

Fig. 1.8 Bird's eye view of rotating armature. Note thumbscrew for fine adjustment

longitudinally along the axon with each depolarization. In a realistic way, the essential participation of electricity in nerve conduction seemed compatible with their dramatically disparate velocities (Fig. 1.10).

Bernstein's theory explained "animal electricity's," down-to-earth conduction velocity, and suggested the all-or-none nature of nerve depolarization and the refractory period.

Galvani had recognized that a certain stimulus strength was required to elicit signal transmission, and that above a certain magnitude, no further response was elicited. This was demonstrated subsequently by Matteuci and in other ways, largely within cardiac muscle. These and other observations led to the "all or nothing" principle formulated by Keith Lucas. This idea arose from observations that after a certain threshold, the size of a contraction stayed constant, no matter how much more stimulus was applied, but until that threshold was reached, no contraction was observed [6]. An exception to that, though, was seemingly found in striated muscle in which increased stimulation *did* lead to increased contraction.

In1905, Lucas showed that increased muscular responses occurred digitally, in discrete steps, pointing toward the concept of muscular fiber recruitment [6]. The increased response was not due to individual fibers responding to higher currents,

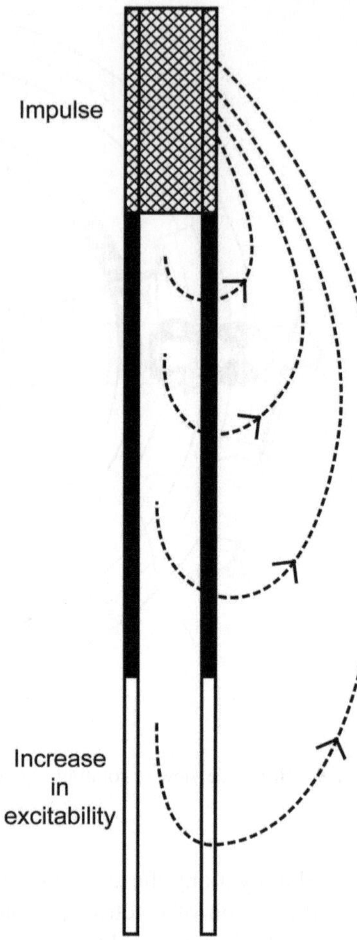

Fig. 1.9 Ludimar Von Hermann's theory of neuronal transmission. This accounted for the comparative sluggishness of nerve conduction; the fast electrical activity was *across* the nerve membrane; forward movement required slower induction

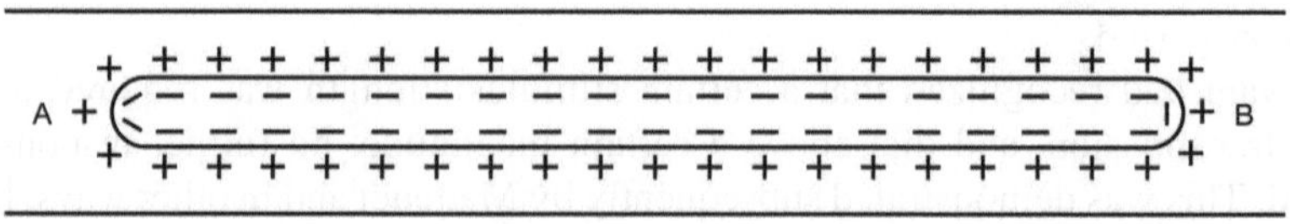

Fig. 1.10 Bernstein's idea of the nerve cell membrane as a variably permeable capacitor

but because *more* fibers were responding: "all or nothing" remained a viable principle (Fig. 1.11).

Through cooling different lengths of neurons to reduce conduction, Lucas and Adrian conceived of a "local energetics" principle responsible for nerve propagation. They compared this to a trail of gunpowder leading to an explosive keg;

Fig. 1.11 Lucas elegantly demonstrated the uniform nature of nerve depolarization, and its overshoot of mere neutrality, and critical elements of the modern theory of differential neuronal membrane permeability. If the neuronal membrane simply lost all resistance, the depolarization would fall to the baseline, not beyond

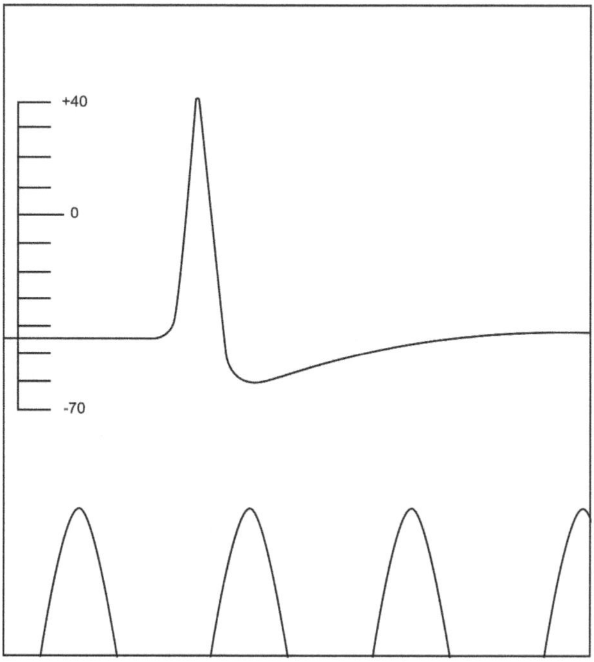

lighting one end of the trail resulted in a propagation of fire traveling the distance to the keg.

> ... If a small portion of gunpowder is wetted in the middle of the train, it will take a longer time for the fire to reach the keg, as some of the energy will go towards evaporating the water in the trail before proceeded along. That will take some time, slowing the movement down, but the speed will resume once the dry powder is again reached; the propagation down this trail is re-energized by a property of the material locally. If a long area of gunpowder is slightly wetted, or a short area made so wet that there is insufficient heat to totally evaporate the contained water, the energy from the propagating fire will be exhausted before reaching the keg, and no explosion will occur ... [6, 11].

Nerve conduction was then viewed in a similar way—as a propagated disturbance resulting at least in part from local energetics, properties of the nerve, not the stimulus applied to it. The cooling of small areas supported this idea. The temperature dependence of the signal suggested a chemical process. Other observations, noting that multiple subthreshold stimuli can sum to achieve depolarization, and that there is a refractory phase following depolarization, suggested some local regenerative process.

Negative neuronal stimulation functioned exactly like an electric current in a wire, but positive stimulation, in which positive ions entered the cell and depolarized it, made for transmembrane migration of positive ions into the cell—exactly the opposite of what would be expected if the membrane were not actively maintaining the charge differential. This characterized the membrane as an active, electrical mechanism that explained the all or nothing rule, the refractory period, and the fact that there is a threshold for triggering the impulse. It also explained in more detail why nerve conduction is so much slower than the electricity that powers it and its temperature-dependence: nerve conduction was seen as an organic process subject to variation with the speeds of metabolism.

In the 1950s, electrophysiology re-entered the sea. Thanks to two pairs of British researchers and a few giant squid, the world better understood the way an electrical impulse (or action potential) is generated. Alan Hodgkin and Andrew Huxley of Cambridge University conducted a series of experiments that inserted tiny microelectrodes into the axon of a giant squid (perfect for electrophysiological recordings due to its sheer size) and were able to measure the membrane voltage changes both during an action potential and at rest. They found a positive potential outside and a negative potential of about 50 mV inside the cell, an "overshoot" beyond mere neutrality at the time of depolarization, and definitively documented the simultaneous progression of the action potential and nerve impulse conduction along the axon [6].

It was only a short time before it was seen that this resting potential was the "animal electricity" postulated by Galvani, which a submaximal stimulus would promote and a supramaximal stimulus would evoke. Bernstein's theory, while an essential scaffold for constructing the modern theory, wrongly held that the membrane would become permeable to any ion movements during depolarization, though the overshoot in his own actual recordings suggest otherwise (see Fig. 1.7).

Hodgkin and Huxley also showed an increased local excitability beyond a region of blocked conduction. In 1949 they showed that the action potential changed with Na concentration [6], suggesting that the action potential was due to Na permeability, while the resting potential was due to K permeability of the membrane. This mechanism also explained the "overshoot" that Bernstein and others had recorded. If the transmembrane potential were equally permeable to all ions, the action potential would go to zero with depolarization. However, the action potential actually overshot in the other direction, rendering the inside positive with respect to outside [6]. If membrane permeability were increased only to Na, this overshoot could be explained ... but still difficult to prove.

Accurate and precise measurement of the electrical events surrounding an action potential was exceedingly difficult at the time due to rapid and overlapping explosive and regenerative (depolarizing and repolarizing) components of the event. This obscured the permeabilities of the membrane to ions that, as it later turned out, were voltage dependent and different from moiety to moiety, changing every fraction of a millisecond that one studied the action potential duration [6].

The technology that helped to clarify the processes was introduced in 1949 by Cole and Marmot. Their technique allows the generation and maintenance of a constant voltage—a "voltage clamp"—allowing the ion flows and permeabilities of a cell to be accurately measured without the difficulties described above [6]. From this evolved the current understanding of transmembrane potential differences maintained by active ionic transport and dynamic voltage-dependent differentials in ionic permeabilities. These appeared to be due to the electric fields generated by the ion currents, resulting in depolarization thresholds and conduction down nerve fibers, ultimately stimulating muscular contraction via changing electrical potentials and the release of neurotransmitters that they induce [6].

The mechanisms of this transport and the differential permeabilities have not been worked out fully, but the framework developed 60 years ago is largely the one that persists today. The basics of differential membrane permeability are strongly supported by the fact that sodium current is uniquely blocked by tetrodotoxin (of the puffer fish) and the potassium current by tetraethylammonium.

With these discoveries electrophysiology consistently linked with physics and chemistry. Measurement of sodium, calcium, potassium, and increasingly more complex organic compounds has revealed electrophysiological phenomena that were compatible and indeed sensitive to well-understood chemical and physical principles. The doors to creative investigation swung open significantly more widely. The last 50 years have witnessed a fabulous extension of our abilities to examine ourselves. From listening for breath sounds and feeling the pulse, we have developed a truly vast array of chemical and physical—electronic and optical—assays of the human condition. Furthermore, based largely on the consistent application of physical and chemical laws in biology, we have innovated genetic means to understand that most challenging of organisms, ourselves. From immunoelectrophoresis and nanogram analyses to neural scans and gene therapy, electricity plays as important a part in Medicine as it does in communication and industry.

EMG Specific Advances

In the late 1800s and early 1900s, the invention of the cathode ray tube vastly improved existing EMG technology. In 1905, photography was added to the machine to record its luminescent tracings. The tube was hardened in 1912 enabling its use with higher voltages, supporting higher amplification requirements (though a patent was not granted until 1925, so the use was restricted) [1].

In 1911, Cluzet employed a battery of condensers in clinical electrodiagnosis. However, the EMG technology chiefly measured chronaxie, the clinical relevance of which was open to serious question [1]. The concept was generally felt to be sound, but the techniques were labor intensive, time consuming, and yielded only generalizations.

During and after World War I, chronaxie was still being studied in laboratories, but was being abandoned with equal zeal in hospitals. At a time when medical facilities were inundated with wounded soldiers and civilians, institutions lacked the time and personnel to perform these laborious tests. By the Second World War, however, the technology had improved enough to be quite useful for the peripheral nerve injuries turning up in hospitals [1].

Forbes and Thacher used the electron tube (CRT) in 1920 to amplify action currents in conjunction with the string galvanometer, getting good action potential, and motor unit recordings. They probably were the first to use floating electrodes on a moving body. They were famously able to record EMG signals in elephants [1].

A couple of years later, Gasser and Erlanger swapped the galvanometer for the cathode ray oscilloscope. Although they were only able to glean rough information due to the stochastic nature of the myoelectric signal, these techniques anticipated future EMG equipment [1]. The technology for signal detecting improved steadily from 1930 to 1950.

In 1929, Adrian and Bronk developed the coaxial/concentric needle electrode, measuring potentials from a single muscle fiber as opposed to averaging potentials from many. Adrian also added audio to the device, so data could be picked up by ear as well as by sight [1].

Clinical knowledge advanced in the 1930s and 1940s. In 1935, tracings from patients with myasthenia gravis showed motor neuron amplitude fluctuations. Three years later tracings made on bromide paper allowed differentiation between fasciculation and fibrillation. In 1941, characteristic potentials of myotonia were recorded, and EMG validated findings in muscular atrophy. Rhythmic potentials in rigid muscles at rest were identified in Parkonsonian patients. The monopolar needle electrode was developed by Herbert Jasper in 1944, which he used to do groundbreaking research with epilepsy [1].

Circa the 1930s, EMGs generally consisted of comparing the laboratory findings with "normal" muscle potentials. In 1944, Weddell, Feinstein, and Pattle published a complete report of EMG to date in what became an early standardization reference manual for researchers and clinicians. Before that, EMG was difficult to use clinically: the instruments were custom-built and expensive; the procedures disorganized and non-standard. The manual outlined normal muscle potentials and presented common neuromuscular entities [1]. As such, it was an invaluable tool to expanding the use of EMG. Though in 1944 only a few specialists had ever used an EMG, by 1950, EMG technology was all but required for any reputable physical medicine department.

John Basmajian compiled what was known in EMG again in 1962, which further consolidated and standardized its usage, rendering reporting more uniform. In 1965 he founded ISEK (the International Society of Electrophysiological Kinesiology) for precisely this purpose. Basmajian also created a fine-wired electrode which was more durable and more comfortable than its predecessors [1].

But in spite of Herculean efforts to stabilize and delimit the field, creativity broke loose again. In 1966, Hardyck used surface EMG to detect new specific disorders that were previously unclassified and alas, unincluded in Basmajian's work. Cram and Steger introduced a clinical method for scanning a variety of muscles using other EMG sensing devices in the early 1980s.

Batch production of necessarily small, lightweight instruments and amplifiers began in the mid-1980s, as integration techniques in electrodes advanced. Electrodiagnostics, as we know it, requires standard instruments and standard practices: a matching pair. Certainly electrodiagnosis has always required that the patient hold still. Against this constant background, deviations from normal, pathological, or just idiosyncratic, could be measured and evaluated. Given its broad consistency with organic and inorganic chemistry, and many aspects of physics, from entropy measurements to electronics, contemporary electrodiagnosis is both hard science and based on cooperation between patient and examiner: exquisitely applicable to the curious biological beings that make up humankind. A broad assortment of impressive experiments reported over hundreds of years by thousands of investigators has been brought to bear on individuals' unique problems.

There may be no better way to put our current practice into perspective than to assess how we use it in examining our patients. Revisiting the physical examination itself, the fundamental and historic diagnostic activity, may help fully to appreciate the place and playbill of NCV and EMG in contemporary Medicine. It is to this interface between *medical knowledge* with *what is wrong with the patient* to which we now must turn.

References

1. Kite, C. "Annual Report." *Humane Soc.* 1774;31–32.
2. Schechter, DC. "Origins of Electrotherapy I." *N Y State J Med.* 1971;997–1007.
3. Pain Management Technologies. "Tens Unit Therapy for Pain Free Pain Relief." 2002. http://www.paintechnology.com/051.htm
4. Piccolino, M. "Luigi Galvani and animal electricity: two centuries after the foun- dation of electrophysiology." *Trends Neurosci.* 1997;20(10):443–8.
5. Du Bois-Reymond, E. *Untersuchungen uber thierische Elektricitat.* Reimer, Berlin, 1848.
6. Licht, Sidney, ed. *Electrodiagnosis and Electromyography.* Waverly Press Inc, Baltimore, 1961.
7. Piccolino., M. "Animal electricity and the birth of electrophysiology: the legacy of Luigi Galvani." *Brain Res Bull.* 1998;46(5):381–407.
8. Arezzo, Francesco Redi of. *Experiments in the Generation of Insects.* Trans. Mab Bigelow. Chicago: Open Court, n.d.
9. Cajavilca, C, Varon, J, Sternbach, GL. "Luigi Galvani and the foundations of electrophysiology." *Resuscitation.* 2009;80(2):159–62.
10. Schechter, DC. "Origins of Electrotherapy II." *N Y State J Med.* 1971;1114–24.
11. Schuetze, SM. "The discovery of the action potential." *Trends Neurosci.* 1983;6:164–68.

Chapter 2
Electrodiagnosis and the Physical Examination: Casting a Fine Net Widely

"EMG extends the clinical examination"—But to what extent?

Abstract The history of electrodiagnosis displays a mutual dependence on understanding in physics and chemistry as well as in anatomy and histology. The confluence of these knowledge makes up the strength and reliability of the physical examination. This chapter offers a framework in which innovations in the clinical examination and the distinction between provocative and evocative maneuvers in the electrophysiological examination may be evaluated.

Keywords Vitalists · Interactive · Physical examination · Signs · Symptoms · Evocative maneuver · Provocative maneuver · AANEM · Standardization · Specificity · Sensitivity · Pathognomonic

When it was understood that plants grow from seeds, plants became domesticated and agriculture began. When people realized the electrochemical basis of nerve transmission, electrophysiology was born. As the history we have just reviewed demonstrates, electricity was applied as medical treatment for a good many centuries before it came to any diagnostic use. Only after the electrical component of our physiology became understood, could electrodiagnostics have any diagnostic application; just as blood flow must be understood before cardiac auscultation can realistically influence diagnosis.

Summary of the First Chapter and Perspective on the Next

Unsurprisingly, electricity caught human attention due to its effect on us. Soon that attention was focused on how our organisms employ it, and with the Enlightenment as fulcrum, it has catapulted into one of our foremost instruments for self-study: it is recognized as a basic element in animal physiology. Not only EMG but also ECG, EEG, and ENG evoked potentials of every kind record and interpret the "animal electricity" inherent in biological processes. This springs from the work of Galvani. To varying degrees, all imaging studies, all scans and scopes, and almost every

L.M. Fishman, A.N. Wilkins, *Functional Electromyography*,
DOI 10.1007/978-1-60761-020-5_2, © Springer Science+Business Media, LLC 2011

diagnostic device beyond a stethoscope and a reflex hammer, and a tape measure employ the electromagnetic spectrum. This we may trace back to Volta.

As was noted about the late eighteenth Century, "... the most striking similarity between electricity and "the nervous principle" was that very little was known about either" [1]. But this naivety ran straight into the Age of Enlightenment, just as it had gained fearsome momentum. We can possibly trace the origin of the antagonistic relationship between the "vitalists" and the scientists back to the medieval view of Life as divine in origin and therefore inscrutable. This may have been a remnant of the Middle Ages that erroneously revived the controversies between Galvani and Volta. So little was known about electricity that declaring it as basic to live movement might have seemed obscurantist ... and a reference back to what was divinely unknowable: the thunderbolts of the gods. Volta appears to have taken Galvani's approach that way, though actually, the two men were each quite devoted scientists. It may (wrongly) have appeared, during the Enlightenment, that each group was claiming electricity "on their side "—the vitalists asserting that this inexplicable and unknown phenomenon was, like the soul, unreachable, an indefinable *je ne sais quoi*, and something like sacred; and the scientists asserting that this force was easily generated by any man or woman with a piece of amber and a wheel, and might well prove to be as un-spiritual as carbon or oxygen.

Some intellectuals of the time might have seen things in this polarized way. But it was not the actual situation: Luigi Galvani, the physician and anatomist, believed electrical phenomena, no more or less than lightning, were basic to animal functioning, as Volta put it, "animal electricity ... a kind of electricity inherently linked to life itself, and intrinsic to some animal functions" [2] while Volta himself felt electricity was strictly an inorganic phenomena. Yet both of their extensive life works are empirical, experimental, and open-minded in so many other ways.

In particular, Galvani was not claiming any mysterious unknowability about electricity. On the contrary, he spent his life trying to learn what he could. The chief difference was that Galvani looked at electrical phenomena as a biologist, while Volta thought, experimented, and wrote like a physicist. Their mutual innocence of the electrochemical and membrane-related events of nerve transmission held them apart.

From our vantage point, both men were profoundly correct, and each actually gave great credence to the other. Volta's battery is really an inorganic reconstruction of the torpedo fish; Galvani's measurements were made with an instrument of magnets and wire. Their controversy seems more a shadow of the musty air of the Middle Ages than in the substance of their mutual inquiry.

Relevance to Our Subject

Subsequent investigation and theories explaining their findings have reconciled these two seminal thinkers: yes, live things generate electrical currents that are essential to their functioning, and yes, in highly complex ways, they still obey the fundamental laws of physics. But in a sense, the polarization of "scientific" or "objective" versus "vital" or "intrinsic to life" still persists in spite of their obvious compatibility. Strict metabolic studies have been seen in contrast to human and animal appetites: B12 injections seem antithetical to cookbooks; signs are carefully differentiated from symptoms, electrophysiological parameters separated from intentional behavior, and body from mind. Yet, contemporary holistic insights incline one in just the opposite direction: you are what you eat, your environment affects the way you feel and behave, including symptoms and signs—functional MRI and event-related-evoked potentials link our very thoughts and perceptions with electrophysiological and vascular events. What you think affects your galvanic skin response, and what you do affects how you feel and what you feel.

Medicine has no current need for amber or the electric eel. Yet in spite of its *therapeutic* antiquity, electro*diagnostic* work dates back only to Du Bois-Reymond and is only 160 years old. We state that "electrodiagnosis is an extension of the physical examination," but the physical examination, like therapeutic use of electricity, goes back thousands of years. Electrodiagnosis has, perhaps, not become fully adapted, not used fully, in extending the physical examination.

Today electrical arrangements are used *therapeutically* more than ever from electroconvulsive therapy and TENS to EMG-operated prosthetic limbs and esophageal speech devices to hearing aids. Each involves understanding human needs and then creating an interface with human electrophysiology to serve them.

Incorporating more "vitalistic," i.e., relevant to actual life considerations in electrophysiological evaluations will only bring more means to bear on our patients' problems. The rest of this book attempts to take a few aspects of the physical examination—used *diagnostically* for many years—and analyze them electrophysiologically, better to understand their pathogenetic mechanisms and devise effective remedies for the conditions they create. We can then use the same electrodiagnostic techniques to document the remedies' efficacy and to design and test better ones.

Developing alongside all types of technological windows into the human body and the soul, with as broad and fanciful a beginning as the first human encounter with amber or the electric fish, has been the use of electrophysiological measures in the physical examination. From earliest times we have made notice of each other and drawn conclusions from our observation: from "Johnny, your lips are blue, you're cold, get out of the water," to the vivid descriptions of people by Jane Austin or Fyodor Dostoyevsky. With electrodiagnostic precision, we can now make just as matter of fact a statement: "Your nerve conductions are all quite slow. You have a neuropathy, let's check your blood sugar."

Today we might say the physical examination has advanced under the skin, with imaging studies that in the case of atomic force microscopy, get inside the bones, functional MRIs that mirror our very processes of thinking and perception, and cardiac stress-testing that measures not just the structure but the behavior of the heart. Still, through the centuries, while physical evidence of pathologic conditions guides more sophisticated inquiry, the motive and procedure are still faithfully reflected in "Get out of the water, Johnny. Your lips are blue." It must apply ultimately to a person's condition, and it must imply, directly or indirectly, its cause and treatment.

The Physical Examination Is Not Just Physical

Essentially, in everything but a perfunctory check-up, the clinician's encounter with a patient is suspicion- or complaint-driven. It focuses on that suspicion or complaint and all future developments spring from it, sometimes in a linear fashion and sometimes surprisingly. There is the time during which the physician or therapist is passive and the patient is active, in which the patient gives, either in writing or in speech, the reason for the first visit. Even at that time, the physician or other clinician starts thinking: what is this like, have I seen it or read about it, or what does it sort of resemble, but not quite?

But symptoms are more sensitive than specific, and there is usually some question about which of a number of pathogenetic processes are causing the patient's suffering. And the critical question is "How can we find out?" The order of things to come is cast by those first clinical moments of reckoning, though the way things proceed may depend on the results of the first probings. But is it all probing?

"You Can Observe a Lot Just by Looking."—*Yogi Berra*

It begins as the patient and clinician meet, a time in which the clinician observes all manner of things about the patient, and the patient does nothing special, and is, from the viewpoint of their meeting, totally passive. It often starts with the knock on the door and the patient striding across the office. This of necessity precedes any further doings, but extends throughout the good physical examination: the physician or nurse or therapist keeps open eyes, ears, nose, and mind, and a sensitive touch. Even the knock can tell you a lot.

This first part is the history (which clearly is also part of the physical) and extends right through every patient–physician encounter.

It Takes Two

Then there is the part generally regarded as the physical examination itself, which is, as we have been saying, part a matter of physician observation of a more or less passive patient: features such as body build, rashes, posture. What overlaps and follows this embodies the uniquely human cooperation that constitutes the heart of every physical examination, the part that is interactive. From the patellar reflex to finger-to-nose-to-finger, the patient and physician are in a sort of dance, whether finely choreographed or ad hoc. On the doctor's part it is based on anatomy, physiology, pathology, and a calculating mind that has been to school; from the patient, it springs from trust and the motivation to learn more about what is and is not wrong and get well. Patellar reflex testing may at first appear involuntary but it is interactive: few people would contest that the patient's contribution to the test is critical to its success. Regardless of the presence or absence of the reflex, the patient is duty-bound to remain still, with quadriceps relaxed.

The interactive physical examination, those aspects of the examination that could not be performed by an observant and sophisticated writer or journalist, are those aspects in which "pure" perception is insufficient, the parts supporting and confirming or ruling out diagnoses. They are, taken together, a rational rather than a merely descriptive task. They may be as directly relevant as testing the bicipital strength of a patient complaining of weakness to Dr. House-like examination of the toenails in episodic fainting.

It is basically knowing how different conditions manifest themselves and looking at the patient for the symptoms and signs that indicate them. When the initial probings do not support diagnosis number 1, then one does not completely forget about it but begins to look for the next most likely diagnosis and so on. The physical examination is a suspicion-guided inquiry, like most inquiries, and requires that the examiner think on his or her feet. The process is inductive rather than deductive, and reasoning about the findings may be somewhat discretionary, but reasoning is not optional.

What are the limits of the physical examination? Instruments like stethoscopes are certainly part of the physical examination. Does the standard MRI test anything that is not physical? Are MRIs then extensions of the physical examination? What about a CBC or bone biopsy? More to the point here, to what extent *is* the EMG an extension of the physical examination?

If all the possible elements in a physical examination were put up on a blackboard, it would make a dizzying array: blood pressure, sensation at the first web spaces, are the gonads descended, do the eyes move in conjunction? Looking at it from that perspective, a medical student might wonder where the examination ends and the lab tests begin. But one might consider the physical examination is something that you do in the patient's presence, and requires the patient's consent, if not cooperation. One might classify what takes place in the physical examination according to the predominant agent. Is the patient's activity salient, or the clinician's, or are they both active?

Analyzing from the patients' point of view, we may divide into three separate columns what doctors and patients do. In some aspects of the physical examination, the clinician is much more active than the patient (passive), in some the patient undertakes the predominantly active role (active), and in some it is more or less 50–50 (interactive). Some common physical examination activities would be easy to classify:

Interactive	Patient Active	Clinician Active
Visual acuity	Cardiac stress test	Skin sensory testing
Muscle testing	Gait analysis	EEG
Pulmonary auscultation	Barium swallow	CT scan
Mental status examination	Tests for dysdiadochokinesis	Clubbing, cyanosis

This is often a matter of degree, of emphasis. Clinicians' activity (or equipment they employ) is essential to muscle testing, but the patient puts in some critical effort too. Cardiac stress testing equipment has to function, but it basically just records rather than reacting: the patient does most of the work. Therefore, the patient is more the active ingredient in cardiac stress testing, while muscle testing is interactive. People cannot do much at the time to alter a sleep-EEG; therefore, we would have to say that the patient is rather spectacularly passive in that situation. But both the patient and the clinician have to take part in any case.

Veterinarians do use stethoscopes without instructions to the creatures they examine, but human patients cooperate when physicians or nurses listen for the lungs' sounds. Patients had better volunteer whether the pinwheel feels the same at the left shin as the right, but their activity in sensory testing may be limited to just that. The categories given here may have grey edges; nevertheless, as a matter of emphasis, the drift of this tripartite division may be clear by now.

Within this triage, parts of the EMG examination as commonly performed today are of necessity interactive. Determining the findings with partial patient effort and seeking full interference patterns absolutely require patient involvement. Occasionally, by the time needle-testing gets up to the biceps or triceps, patients may pose the question, "Couldn't this test be done under anaesthesia?" and the inevitable answer is "No." Spontaneous activity might be isolated during sleep, but other parts of the needle examination require a conscious patient and definite cooperation. In the succeeding chapters, we propose further patient involvement, chiefly in nerve conduction and H-reflex studies.

Electromyography is a powerful diagnostic tool to evaluate the function and the many dysfunctions of the peripheral nervous system exactly because EMG evaluation serves as a direct extension of the physical examination. It must be taken in that context to be maximally accurate and effective. There are virtually no single wave forms that are pathognomonic of specific disease entities. Rather, there are patterns in the data. Careful history taking and neurological evaluation lead to a differential diagnosis, doing the groundwork for the electrodiagnostics. In this way, electrodiagnosis for each condition is different and at times must be tailored to specific needs and questions that arise in a given patient's assessment.

While symptoms often suggest a great many more diagnoses than are present, and EMG may winnow the list down to a few viable alternatives, the opposite is also true: [3] found a relatively high proportion of individuals who had normal physical examinations and abnormal electrodiagnostic studies. This has been found in MRI examination of the lumbar spine as well [4]. But that is just the point. When MRI finds two different structural anomalies, say, spinal stenosis and herniated nucleus pulposis compressing an exiting root, both at L4-5, one wants to know which is causing the patient's pain! This is where particular maneuvers might help us.

To understand how we do this requires a further distinction: between those aspects of the physical examination that observe or measure what is already present, such as heart rate and temperature, and those that seek to bring out latent features, such as cold calorics or the Hoffmann test: tendencies or propensities that may be quite informative, important, or dangerous, yet are not manifestly present, but rather lurking within the patient's makeup nonetheless. Examples of what is manifestly present at the moment of the examination, and need only be detected, would be positive sharp waves indicating denervation or jitter. Examples of what is latent, but can be brought out are signs of muscle fatigue by repetitive stimulation in myasthenia gravis or H-reflex enhancement through the Jendrassik maneuver.

We can distinguish between those maneuvers that *bring out, enhance, or evoke* a state of affairs that is currently present but undetectable, such as weakness enhanced by repeated effort or mild spasticity, from those maneuvers that *cause to exist* or *provoke* conditions that are liable to occur but are more liabilities than actualities. These conditions are latent but would not be present at the time of the examination, unless they were brought about by a maneuver.

We can separate those conditions that need enhancement to be detected, or evoked, from those to which the patient is vulnerable, that are not present, but must be provoked. In order to do this we should first separate out *evocative* maneuvers from *provocative* maneuvers as found in the general physical examination.

Evocative maneuvers	What they evoke
Deep breath in pulmonary auscultation	Râles, sounds of pulmonary edema
McMurray test	Pop indicating medial meniscal tear
Hoffmann test	Hoffmann sign suggests spasticity

None of these maneuvers produces anything beyond a response. There are no cases of deep breaths causing pulmonary edema nor of the McMurray or Hoffmann tests bringing about a medial meniscal tear or spasticity. Evocative maneuvers frequently bring out benign and reassuring features of the patient and are frequently useful to rule out diagnoses. Nevertheless, the presence of rales, the occurrence of a pop, and the flexion of adjacent fingers indicate pathology. The nature of these tests is to reveal what is already there at the moment, but is too faint or inaccessible to be observed directly.

There are evocative maneuvers in electrodiagnosis and are as follows:

Evocative maneuvers in EMG	What they evoke in EMG
Jendrassik	Faint but extant H reflex
Partial patient effort	Recruitment pattern
Maximal patient effort	Full recruitment capacity
Repetitive stimulation	Diminishing muscular response

The reflexes are what they are; the recruitment patterns are there, nerve conduction velocity is, under standard conditions, unvarying, but these things need special conditions such as electrical stimuli and sensitive measurement to be observed. The techniques bring out and amplify, image, and in some way measure or "capture" what is present but otherwise difficult to verify. Evocative maneuvers bring something out that is there anyway.

But evocative maneuvers contrast with provocative maneuvers, which bring about a pathological sign or symptom (or fail to bring it about) that is not present at the time, bur rather is incipient, or latent, or sometimes present, but not extant at the time of the examination. They bring something about, and unlike merely evocative maneuvers, which exemplify or picture something that may or may not be pathological, what provocative maneuvers produce (or fail to produce) is always pathological.

Provocative maneuvers	What they provoke
Cardiac stress test	Ischemia, arrhythmias
Empty can test	Pain
Tensilon test	Weakness

There are very many evocative and provocative tests in contemporary Medicine, from arthrograms (evocative) to the Gaenslen maneuver (provocative). There are some provocative maneuvers in electrodiagnosis as well:

Provocative maneuvers in EMG	What they provoke in EMG
Repetitive stimulation	Reduced CMAP
But there are not many.	

In the rest of this book, we will introduce and attempt to demonstrate the validity of three provocative maneuvers which may be helpful for the clinician, and may further illustrate a valid method for devising other provocative maneuvers in the clinical context as the need for them arises.

Proposed Provocative Maneuvers in Electrodiagnosis

New provocative maneuver	What it provokes	What it means
FAIR test	Delay in H reflex	Sciatic entrapment
Allen test	Delay in PML	Thoracic outlet syndrome
3-min extension	Delay in H reflex	Positional lumbar stenosis

Subsequent chapters will present the case for each one of these maneuvers: the theoretical justification, the practical ways and means of performing them, and the outcome of using these results in treating patients.

Philosophical Reflection of the Yet Unseen

The history of electricity in Medicine from Chapter 1 traces a path toward standardization. Weddell, Feinstein, and Pattle's [5–7] reference manual for researchers and clinicians in 1944 brought a reasonably well-accepted norm that presented a standard for organizing and comparing the practices of a previously heterogeneous assortment of practitioners. Perhaps more to the point, a reference point enabled practitioners if not to establish, then at least to estimate what was normal, what constituted deviations from normal, and what medical conditions were associated with which departures from normal.

Standardization was exactly what was needed in a field born of controversy. From its groping origins, electrophysiology and the study of electricity itself floundered in the dark to learn fundamental truths, the basic behavior of the phenomena at hand from which experimental evidence could be evaluated and understood. Like any science, electrophysiology and indeed the physics of electricity had to establish a concensus before a body of accepted work could grow.

At first there were finely reported but roughly constructed reports on phenomena with torpedo fish, lightning, and frogs. Soon thereafter were experiments with materials and measurements of speed and force, connection with physics, another science in which metrics already existed. Then finer measurements ensued, and with Bernstein, a working theory that fit most of the facts and reconciled some of the apparent contradictions with physics. As familiarity with the phenomena increased, and a tantalizing flurry of speculation about what was going on proliferated, there developed a good deal of near-chaotic investigation and reporting. This led in a Hegelian progression of "thesis–antithesis-synthesis" to a disseminated and accepted compilation of standard procedures and normal values for tests, using straightforward parameters such as millivolts and meters per second. In less than 10 years following Weddell, Feinstein and Pattle's publication, electrodiagnosis grew from a practice that could be considered either exotic diagnostic work or clinical research to a requirement in every department of Physical Medicine and Rehabilitation by 1950.

Like any group of scientists, believing that there is a truth, electrodiagnosticians aimed to advance toward more universal standards of practice, a better measurement of normal, and tighter and tighter margins of error.

John Basmajian's ISEK (the International Society of Electrophysiological Kinesiology), created in 1965, is illustrative of these motives [8]. The later work of Jun Kimura and many others, and the AANEM itself reflect the same goals and themes [9–11]. Compendious volumes and practical handbooks are indispensible for any broad-based human endeavor intended to find truth through the efforts of many researchers and a broad body of work

But in a vital, advancing field, this uniformity must be the basis of further experimentation, a firm basis from which to launch new forays into unknown territory. The standards of practice must function as unvarying paradigms from which innovations can be objectively judged, but they cannot be used to stifle curiosity, and discourage experimentation which is, by its very nature, less certain in its conclusions. No established work, like a rock foundation, should support efforts at innovation as only it can.

We ask the reader to suspend judgment while examining what we are about to present. Although it definitely has precedent in the evolution of electrodiagnosis, it is new and represents a departure from what is well established using those very well-established principles and values as a guide. As electrodiagnosis is an extension of the physical examination, electrophysiological measurement in provocative maneuvers is presented as an extension of EMG.

We will introduce these maneuvers one by one, and after describing how we have implemented each of them, and the results, we will produce what evidence we can of their clinical utility.

There is another matter that we must consider first, in order to appreciate the need that the first two of these provocative maneuvers fill, that renders these provocative maneuvers more valuable than they might seem to be otherwise. It is to this that we must now turn.

References

1. Schuetze, SM. "The discovery of the action potential." TINS, May, 1983.
2. Piccolino, M. "Animal electricity and the birth of electrophysiology: the legacy of Luigi Galvani." *Brain Res Bull.* 1998;46(July 15 (5):381–407.
3. Lauder, TD, Dillingham, TR, Andary, M, Kumar, S, Pezzin, LE, Stephens, RT, Shannon, S. "Predicting electrodiagnostic outcome in patients with upper limb symptoms: are the history and physical examination helpful?". *Arch Phys MedRehabil.* 2000;81:436–41.
4. Jensen, MC, Brant-Zawadzki, MN, Obuchowski, N, Modic, MT, Malkasian, D, Ross, J. "Magnetic resonance imaging of the lumbar spine in people without back pain." *NEJM.* 1994;331:69–73.
5. Schechter, DC. "Origins of Electrotherapy I." *N.Y. State J. Med.* 1971;71:997–1007.
6. Schechter DC. "Origins of Electrotherapy II." *N.Y. State J. Med.* 1971;71:1114–1124.
7. Licht, S, Ed. Electrodiagnosis and Electromyography. Waverly Press Inc, Baltimore, 1961.
8. Basmajian, JV. "Electromyography Comes of Age." *Science.* 1972 May 12;176(4035):603–9.
9. Kimura, J. 2001. *Electrodiagnosis in Diseases of Nerve and Muscle: Principles and Practice.* Oxford University Press.
10. Perotto, AO, Delagi, EF, Iazetti, J, Morrison, D. 2005. *Anatomical Guide For The Electromyographer: The Limbs And Trunk.* Springer.
11. Braddom, RI, Johnson, EW. "Standardization of H reflex and diagnostic use in S1 radiculopathies." *Arch Phys Med Rehabil.* 1974;55:161–66.

Chapter 3
Dynamic Electrodiagnosis: Provocative/Evocative Maneuvers Define Diagnoses of Exclusion and Refine Dual Diagnoses

Abstract In this chapter, we introduce the three diagnoses we shall discuss hereafter. We proceed to sketch out the current wisdom on these subjects, and delineate our strategies for going forward. Since two of the diagnoses we are approaching are currently diagnoses of exclusion, we begin with the logical untenability of that concept.

Keywords Diagnosis of exclusion · Differential diagnosis · Adson's maneuver · Allen test · Hallstead maneuver · Thoracic outlet syndrome · Neurologic thoracic outlet syndrome · Spinal stenosis · Brachial plexus · Electromyographer · Brachial plexus · Proximal motor latency · F wave · H reflex · Functional electrodiagnostics · Reversible prolongation · Radiculopathy · Spondylolisthesis · Pancoast tumor · Piriformis syndrome · Entrapment · Neural scan · Botulinum neurotoxin · FAIR test

The Fallacy Inherent in a "Diagnosis of Exclusion"

Differential diagnosis stands at the heart of the last 2 years of medical school. What physician cannot remember a hospital-based luminary chalking up a dozen or more possibilities for a given symptom set? Usually it is an infectious disease specialist: "A 37-year-old woman with joint pain, pulmonary nodules and a rash?"

"It could be rheumatoid arthritis, breast cancer, sarcoidosis, MRSA, tuberculosis, chicken pox pneumonia, small cell carcinoma, gonorrhea, a drug reaction, lupus, psoriatic arthritis, various types of lymphoma or immune deficiency syndromes, syphilis,. . ." and so on.

Then the learned one crosses out the candidates in serial fashion: "But the rheumatoid factor has been negative three times, and the films of the joints show no deterioration; mammograms and even the biopsy were flatly negative;. . ." And sure enough, there is one prime suspect at the end of this useful exercise, and the one left standing turns out, more often than not, to be the villain.

Infectious disease is like that. In fact, the very words "infectious disease" imply that there is a source, vector, a fomite, a pathogen, a single identifiable cause of what

L.M. Fishman, A.N. Wilkins, *Functional Electromyography*,
DOI 10.1007/978-1-60761-020-5_3,

ails the patient. Assembling the likely suspects and then knocking them down one by one give a general location of the patient's condition in the many dimensions of human pathology, and also lend a fair bit of confidence, a sense of precision, and certainty to the eventual diagnosis the process yields.

But what happens when there is no light at the end of the labyrinth? What if all the listed diagnoses get ruled out? That is when the attending physician pulls a rabbit out of his or her hat, and says something like: "there is another diagnosis, of somewhat disputed certitude, that nevertheless seems to fit the symptoms, and [because there are no known strong indications against it, nor, of course, any tests that confirm it] might just be what's going on here." Enter the diagnosis of exclusion.

In a sense, the diagnosis of exclusion is the empirical counterpart of what is called "indirect proof" in mathematics. One shows that all the alternatives to a given theorem lead to something false and therefore the theorem must be true. The analogy appeals to us when we have found all our other explanations fall short, but not our belief that there is an explanation. Unfortunately, in an empirical subject such as medicine, one never, never knows all the alternatives. What clinician would not nod his or her head with Shakespeare's "There is more in this world than you have dreamt of in your philosophies?"

You might call it a working hypothesis. In the case of the 37-year-old woman, maybe it is [let's make one up] Boston fever, exposure to poison ivy, and the flu.

So instead of treating her with chemotherapy after a lumpectomy, as one might do for breast cancer, if it were detected, and not ruled out, we will give her topical steroids and wait, things that would be just wrong with MRSA. We will operate on this hypothesis, the supposition that she has poison ivy and flu, until either the woman's condition improves or some other diagnosis declares itself.

The assumption is, naturally, that one would never look for Boston fever unless nothing else checks out. No one in their right mind would start out looking for a "diagnosis of disrepute," and no one would go slumming along the borders of the medical establishment when a perfectly fine diagnostic entity was already proven!

But something tricky has happened in our thinking here. An assumption has crept in that needs to be ushered out. Sketchy or not, with definitive tests or without them, if a condition *exists*, then it can *coexist* with other conditions. Infectious disease, to take one example, generally looks for *the* cause of a fever, or a swelling, but one could have pneumonia and dehydration, swine flu and syphilis, or a boil on top of a bruise.

Suppose, just for the moment, something false: that the connection between *Rhus radicans* and rash were just suspected. Then once we had ruled out contact dermatitis of the usual types, eczema, psoriasis, and the others in the illustration below, we might hit upon the possibility of a rash being due to exposure to poison ivy...a diagnosis of exclusion (Fig. 3.1).

Of course, as we know today, there is a strong relationship between brushing your skin up against the three-leaved plant and developing the characteristic rash. We also know that you could have poison ivy and pneumonia, or a fractured humerus or glaucoma at the same time. You might even have two types of dermatitis simultaneously (Fig. 3.2).

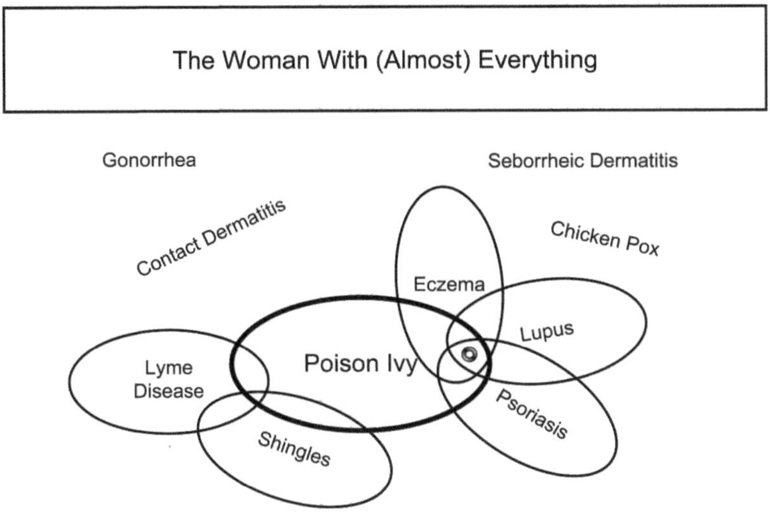

Fig. 3.1 If the state of our knowledge left poison ivy a questionable diagnosis, then excluding the usual suspects in a given situation might strengthen our suspicion that we were confronting a case of it. But if another diagnosis were confirmed, we might very well stop looking

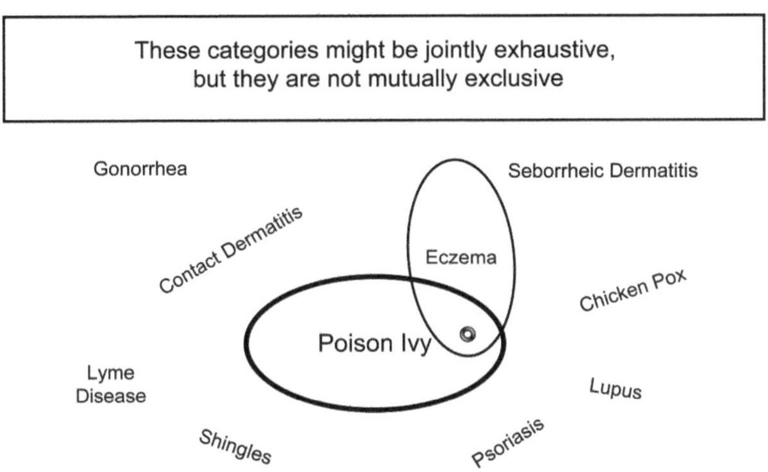

Fig. 3.2 However shaky our information about poison ivy, we could encounter people with it and another skin condition, though we might not know it

One might even encounter the more complex situation in Fig. 3.3.

One could, of course, have a variety of conditions concurrently. Since chronic conditions are by definition cumulative, people tend to have more and more of them as they age. There are mutually exclusive states, such as hyperthermia and hypothermia, or sprained ankle in a double amputation, but in general, for better and for worse, we can and usually do have multiple diagnoses.

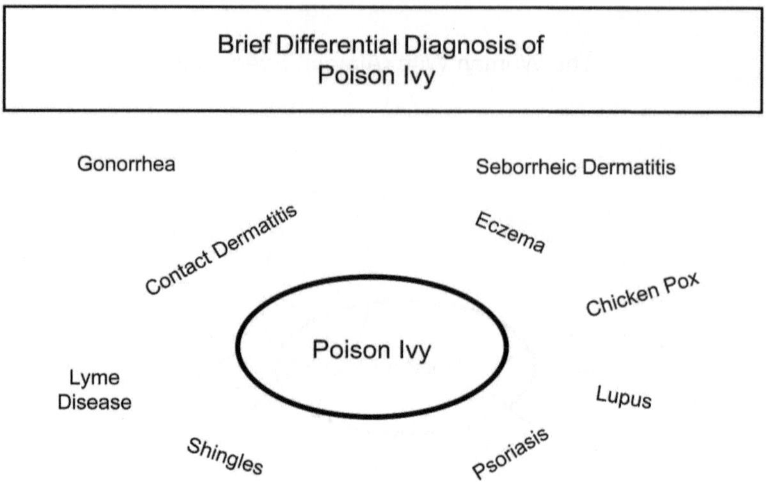

Fig. 3.3 Using a principle of "diagnosis by exclusion" will fail to identify all cases of dual diagnosis

The entity that is a diagnosis of exclusion is therefore necessarily underdiagnosed, for when concurrent with any other diagnosis, it is rarely even mentioned.

One measure of medical progress is the slow conversion of a genuine disease entity from a murky suspicion to a working diagnosis to an identifiable condition. It is at that point that causes can be sought and treatment for the condition evaluated.

Now how does it happen? How does a suspected set of symptoms get a name? One way is through their being noted to occur together and to have something in common. A common cause is one such thing; one reason to lump symptoms together. Asking "what would make exactly this happen?" is how this chapter started, with the differential diagnosis, the search for cause of a set of symptoms.

But there is another reason that symptom-sets end up with a name and are thought of as a diagnostic entity: rheumatoid arthritis has no single known cause, and a wide range of symptoms and signs are attributable to it. The tests, radiological and immunological, and the pathogenetic mechanism are what define the core cases and serve to justify the association of quite a variable group of symptoms with a single diagnosis.

The rest of this book is devoted to tests that may help to identify three other clusters of symptoms that, once assembled, immediately enable one to look for their cause or causes and develop effective treatment. In the first two cases, there has long been a vague sort of examination, a general set of findings that suggests the syndromes, but nothing definitive. The third cluster is too big—occurring where there are too many established diagnoses, and there is no good method to decide how much each of them is contributing to the patient's pain.

The purpose of using an extension of current electrodiagnostic methods is to objectively identify and quantify all three of these conditions by clinically correlating them with the tests' electrophysiological results—something current standard techniques do not accomplish. Dynamic use of electrodiagnosis appears to enable us to do so in a logical and replicable manner. In each case, the electrodiagnostic test is just an extension of the physical examination, just a numerical representation of a physical finding or provocative maneuver that is associated with the condition on which we are focusing.

Thoracic Outlet Syndrome

The cords, divisions, and nerve trunks descending between the scalenus anticus and medius give off their posterior branches and head for the clavicle. The subclavian artery travels upward through the chest and curves sharply downward at the notch in the first rib where it becomes the axillary artery before joining the elements of the brachial plexus, forming a neurovascular bundle that ducks under the clavicle. Subsequently, the nerves and artery (which becomes the brachial artery below the teres minor) run together in that neurovascular bundle beneath the coracoid process in their course to the arm and hand (Fig. 3.4).

Adson's maneuver and its cheiric twin, the Allen test, exploit this relationship. Adson's was originally intended to diagnose a pancoast tumor, which forms at the apex of the lung. In Adson's maneuver, the examiner feels the radial pulse of the suspected arm that has been abducted and externally rotated 90°. The patient is then asked to revolve his or her head 90° ipsilaterally, extend the neck, and take a deep breath. In a positive Adson's maneuver (rotation to affected side) or Allen maneuver (contralateral head rotation), the pulse disappears, ostensibly because an apical mass has exerted a compressive force on the neurovascular bundle that is greater than the patient's systolic blood pressure (Fig. 3.5).

In the course of time, MRI has replaced Adson's maneuver for this type of tumor and for so many others. But by stretching the neurovascular bundle from the cleft between the scalenus anticus and medius to the coracoid process, the maneuver has been thought to be positive in neurological and vascular thoracic outlet syndromes.

Now these two conditions, entrapments of the brachial artery or elements of the brachial plexus, generally at the level of the cords or the proximal sections of the ulnar and median and other nerves that the cords become, are prime examples of "diagnoses of exclusion." As already noted, a positive Adson's maneuver is seen in pancoast tumor, and actually is seen in a fair percentage of asymptomatic shoulders. While it gives some evidence for a position- and respiration-related compression of the neurovascular bundle, a positive Adson's sign is hardly pathognomonic. In fact, since the positive sign reflects only vascular dynamics, it bears no direct relationship to any neurological condition at all. Some cases of tingling and numbness and even weakness in an upper extremity might be vascular in their origin. Adson's maneuver and the Allen test certainly give no evidence to the contrary.

However, there is a way to measure the neurological effect of provocative maneuvers such as these. If any part of the brachial plexus or its immediate projections

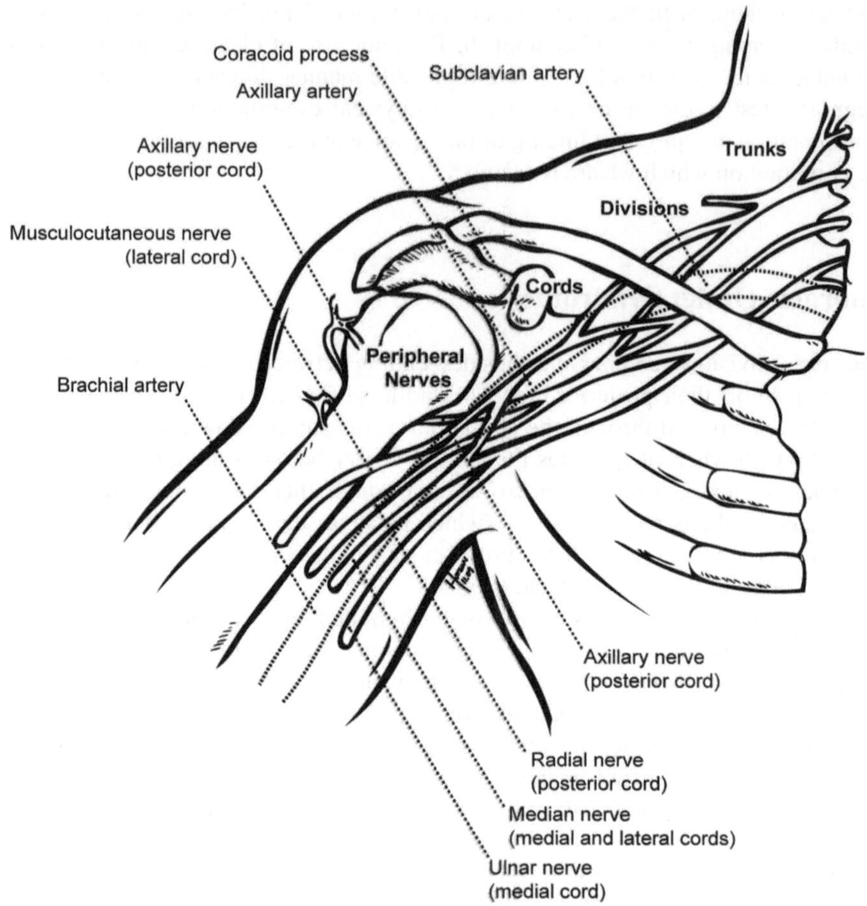

Fig. 3.4 The brachial plexus in its natural habitat

is significantly compressed, that compression ought to slow nerve conduction and possibly also cause some temporal dispersion or conduction block. If this compression is not structural, and is related to any maneuver at all, then it ought to be reversible and relent when the pathological position is released. If the condition occurs frequently or with sufficient intensity, enough to actually damage the neurons, then, of course, it has become structural. This is actually seen in the "zinger" of sports medicine, a forcible and patently unplanned version of Adson's maneuver that takes place on the football field and in bicycle accidents more than elsewhere.

The key to using nerve conduction studies this way is to determine by physical examination what nerve pathways are likely to be involved. Electromyographers are no strangers to this type of deductive process, and it is hardly a problem. Rather, it is an opportunity to graduate "neurological thoracic outlet syndrome" into a distinct

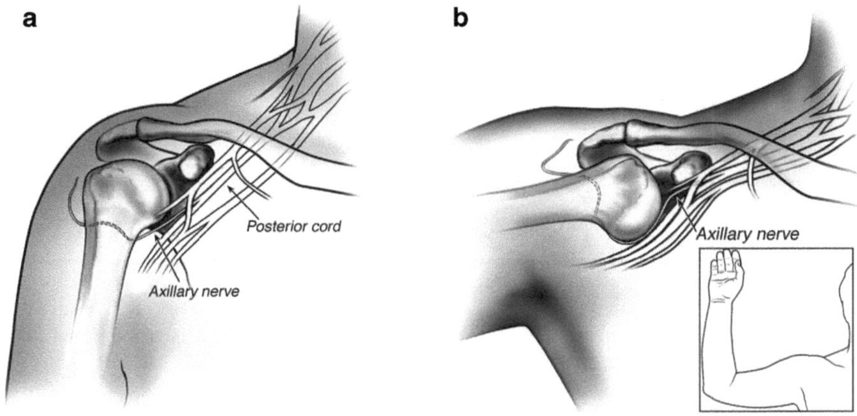

Fig. 3.5 The brachial plexus at rest (**a**) and in Adson's maneuver (ipsilateral head rotation) or the Allen test (contralateral head rotation) (**b**)

entity, no longer a diagnosis of exclusion but rather a condition admitted to the hallowed world of actual diagnoses, able to coexist with radiculopathies, neuropathies and yes, even Pancoast tumors.

Piriformis Syndrome

Piriformis syndrome was long taken to be another diagnosis of exclusion. We were introduced to it by Dr. Steven Ringel, an orthopedic surgeon grasping at straws in the era when CT scans were state-of-the-art: an operating room nurse had severe bilateral sciatica, but no discal pathology, no spinal stenosis, and no other detectible abnormality. The surgeon more or less bursts into the electrodiagnostic lab holding the nurse by the arm, saying the only clue was that she had buttock pain, and added, with a measure of desperation, "may be it is a peripheral entrapment." He shrugged his shoulders and muttered: "like piriformis syndrome." The orthopod did not want to operate simply on the basis of what the patient did not have.

> "There's no test for that," we said.
>
> "Then make one up" he exclaimed, waving one hand in the air as he opened the door with the other, and walked out.

As luck would have it, the first case was bilateral, so there was no comparing one leg with the other. Rather, it was only possible to compare a leg in one position with the same leg in another position, ostensibly one that would tend to intensify the relevant peripheral entrapment. We hypothesized that since the piriformis muscle was an abductor of the thigh, that adduction would stretch it tight, and flexing and internally rotating the thigh would allow us to exert more force through a greater degree of adduction. By flexing the knee as well, we thought we would have better

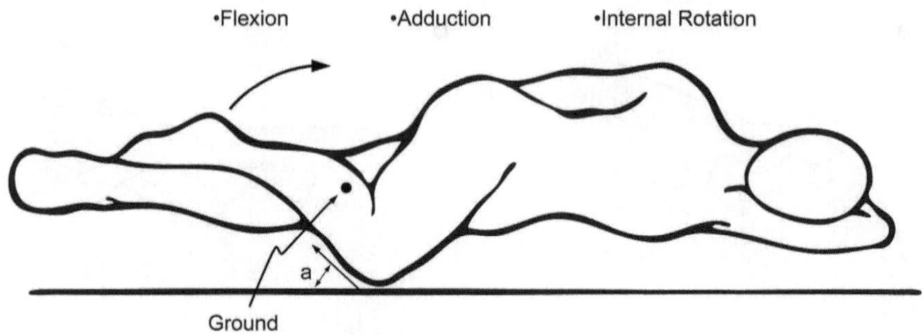

Fig. 3.6 Position for piriformis test. With the knee depressed, the angle α is proportional to the pressure exerted by the muscle on the sciatic nerve

control over what we were doing, since then we could hold down the knee and use the pressure on the lateral ankle to work the muscle with a crank-like motion (Fig. 3.6).

We found a 2-ms prolongation of the H reflex on each side with the maneuver, and repeated it several times, getting very much the same results. We had no controls, but calculated that this was nearly 5 standard deviations beyond the mean for side-to-side variation (S.D. = 0.42 ms), giving us some idea of the magnitude of this replicable change and the unlikelihood of it happening replicably and bilaterally by chance. We also looked at the variably present peroneal H reflexes, since we had little else to go on. They were unchanged by the Flexed, Adducted, Internally Rotated maneuver, which we quickly dubbed the FAIR test.

The EMG was somewhat suggestive. Paraspinals were normal, but there was mild denervation of the gastrocnemius muscles bilaterally, as well as the right flexor digitorum, with increased insertional activity of that same muscle on the left, while all peroneally innnervated muscles, as well as the glutei, hamstrings, and the piriformis muscles themselves were normal. The lack of paraspinal abnormalities suggested that the injury was below the spinal level. The normal EMG findings in the L4-5-S1-S2 muscles whose innervation was through the superior or inferior gluteal nerves, and the hamstrings, whose nerves leave the sciatic trunk before it passes through the sciatic foramen, suggested that the pathology was at or below that level. The bilateral concentration of positive findings to muscles innervated by multiple root levels but only the posterior tibial branch without any abnormalities in the peroneal branch again argued against an intraspinal cause, and located the cause beyond any myotomal organization of the motor nerves, and rather at the level of the sciatic foramen or just beyond. The fact that stretching the piriformis muscle over the sciatic nerve and/or its branches prolonged the posterior tibial H reflexes was gaining significance.

We then looked at the sural sensory nerve amplitudes quite carefully. They were smaller than expected when we compared them with saphenous and ulnar sensory nerves' amplitudes and their relative deviations from "normal" values in various electrodiagnostic texts.

So we had a reasonably compelling picture: normal CT and no paraspinal denervation. A sizeable prolongation of the posterior tibial H reflexes with stretching the piriformis muscle over the sciatic nerve, but otherwise normal values for posterior tibial and peroneal H reflexes bilaterally. No changes in the peroneal H reflex with the same maneuver, and a non-myotomal pattern of denervation of only muscles innervated by the posterior tibial branch of the sciatic nerves. Furthermore, the sural sensory nerve action potentials were small, suggesting a lesion distal to the ganglia.

But it was only a picture.

The physical examination had revealed slight sensory deficit at the dorsal feet and distal lateral calves, buttock tenderness that vaguely reproduced the sciatica, and the history revealed that sitting was worse than any other position. This strengthened the surgeon's resolve, and 2 days later, when the nurse entered his own OR as a patient, we were there, Nikon in our latex-gloved hands.

The operation was short. After gently splitting fibers of the gluteus maximus and clearly identifying the sciatic nerve, Dr. Ringel thinned down the inferior 25% of the piriformis muscle, instilled a little steroid, and closed. We obtained some clear photos of a glistening sciatic nerve that was denuded of vaso nervorum in a 2-cm band just at its intersection with the piriformis muscle. The patient awoke with some incisional pain but no sciatica.

Over the next 7 years, we encountered 34 cases like the OR nurse, and since publishing our method and the results of effective conservative and surgical treatment, have seen upwards of 15,000 patients who were thought to have piriformis syndrome. In our judgment, approximately half of them actually did. But piriformis syndrome has come some distance toward diagnostic independence. Two other methods have lent credence to the diagnosis.

One is diagnostic confirmation by successful treatment. In brief, if the piriformis muscle is responsible for sciatica, then removal, neurolysis, or paralysis of the piriformis muscle ought to relieve the pain. There are a number of studies in which surgical excision or neurolysis has shown high rates of impressive efficacy. Physical therapy, often with injection, and always focused on the muscle, has succeeded in largely alleviating or curing piriformis syndrome in 80% of more than 1,000 cases which we have reviewed carefully [1]. In these cases, the injection sites have been confirmed with EMG, MRI, CT, fluoroscopy, or ultrasound [1–11]. Physical therapy alone has been less persuasive because of its similarity to McKenzie technique and other manual methods applicable to the spine, but has its adherents, current authors included. Together, these studies report more than 2,000 carefully monitored and successfully treated patients.

Other EMG techniques have also been applied successfully for detecting piriformis syndrome [12] (Fig. 3.7).

Neural scans are currently the most effective way to image the soft tissues such as nerves and muscles. Developed and championed by Dr. Aaron Filler at Cedars-Sinai Hospital in Beverly Hills, neural scans essentially take a normal, old-fashioned type of MRI image, and then use digital wizardry to subtract a fat-suppression image from the whole image.

MRI image

—

MRI image without fatty structures

Fatty structures

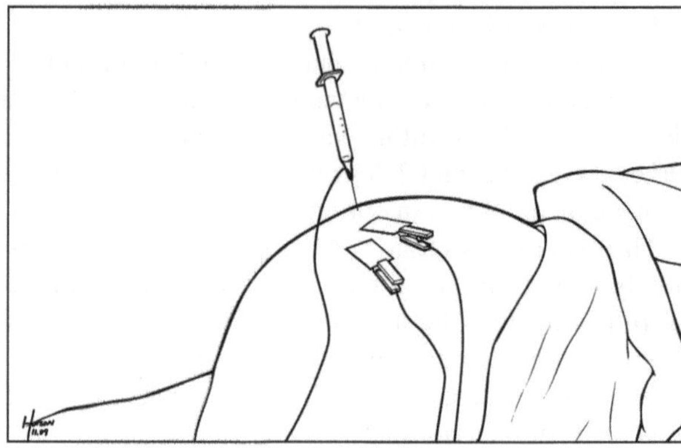

Fig. 3.7 EMG-guided injection into the piriformis muscle

Of course, the fatty myelin sheaths of peripheral nerves render them particularly prominent in the resultant digitally subtracted image. Dr. Filler studied 239 people, approximately half of whom had had unsuccessful spinal surgery, the other half having no conventional MRI evidence of spinal pathology. He used the neural scan to produce hundreds of different images of their spines, lumbosacral plexi, and pelves. Dr. Filler found 67% of these cases of "non-disc" sciatica to be due to piriformis syndrome, but also a small percentage due to far lateral disc herniations and spinal stenoses that were missed, and another 4% due to entrapment of the sciatic nerve at the ischial tunnel. A conventional EMG is likely to pick up paraspinal denervation in a far lateral disc herniation and spinal stenosis, but ischial tunnel versus piriformis syndrome is a distinction that only neural scanning is currently able to make.

Dr. Filler et al., went further. They noted that 1.2 million MRIs were done in 2002 for sciatica, yet only 200,000 surgeries were performed. They concluded that non-disc sciatica may be as common or more common than herniated disc-caused sciatica since fully two-third of these non-disc sciatica appear to be piriformis syndrome [13, 14].

Treatment for piriformis syndrome is persuasively successful. Ours, other physiatrists', neurologists', anesthesiologists', and later Dr. Filler's injection records encourage clinicians to regard piriformis syndrome as a diagnostic entity, since over 80% of people diagnosed with piriformis syndrome and treated by any of these methods have at the very least an extended period of relief. Surgical relief has also been the rule in the small minority of patients requiring it [8–10, 13, 14]. Physical therapy and yoga have helped the vast majority of patients with piriformis syndrome [1, 5, 11, 13–16].

Records from 1976 to 1979 for Olmstead County, Minnesota, which houses the Mayo Clinic, state that piriformis syndrome was diagnosed in 11 of 4,416 cases, giving a diagnostic rate of 0.25%. The quarter century from 1976 to 2001 found 220 cases of piriformis syndrome among 32,655 cases of lower back pain, for a rate of 0.7%, whereas in 2000–2001, the diagnosis was made in 54 of 4,349 cases, yielding a rate of 1.24%, showing nearly 500% rise in that quarter century [17].

There are trends in diagnostics, even fads. In the 1940s, there was anemia or "tired blood." There was a time when lupus erythematosis was blamed for everything, then chronic fatigue, and Epstein–Barr virus. Applying to the entire rogues' gallery of unresolved dilemmas, these diagnoses were, like an erythrocyte sedimentation rate, too broad to have much clinical value. Is it possible that the dictum "sciatica is caused in the spine" has been applied somewhat indiscriminately at times?

Surely this piriformis syndrome is a diagnosis that may be made correctly or withheld incorrectly, like any other. But the point is that currently it appears to be entertained more frequently, yet applied with more discretion since there are tests for it. We intend to show in detail how dynamic electrodiagnosis has been extended to provide these tests for a number of putative diagnoses, and possibly can be extended for more.

Lumbar Spinal Stenosis Versus Herniated Disc

We now leave behind the hazy realm of those phantoms, the diagnoses of exclusion, and enter the courtroom. Diagnoses of exclusion appear where there is no firm diagnosis; here we have the opposite problem: too many accepted diagnoses! The scene is a mystery story, and as the plot unfolds, the question is Who is the culprit? We might need two or three writs of Habeus Corpus: the crime is plain, or rather, usually pain, but there are too many perpetrators. The patient not only has sciatica but also has both spinal stenosis and a herniated disc on MRI, and paraspinal denervation on EMG. Is one or the other responsible? Or is it a conspiracy? If the latter, what proportion of the patient's pain will be relieved by treating one condition, how much by treating the other? The surgeries and the physical therapeutic prescriptions for the two conditions are quite different, whether at the same or different levels. EMG is often useful in identifying each of these conditions, but currently has little value in distinguishing one from the other. The distinction can be very difficult to make, particularly if both conditions occur at the same level, which, as anatomy, trauma, and luck would have it, they frequently do.

In physical therapy the extension maneuvers of the McKenzie technique, for example, are powerfully curative in sciatica due to herniated discs, but relatively contraindicated in lumbar spinal stenosis. Extension has been shown to narrow the already compromised intraspinal canal up to 63% [18–21]. Flexion is beneficial for stenosis but raises the risk of extending a disc's herniation. In surgery, the fusion often needed in stenosis surgeries is a far cry from the simple microdiscectomy that treats many disc herniations. Spondylolisthesis complicates the matter still further, often being a positional variable that gets thrown into the mix: is stenosis more pathological in extension due to spondylolisthesis causing further narrowing in that position?

H reflexes done in different positions can aid the standard EMG examination here. We have compared H reflexes in the anatomical position with those seen in 3-min extension to suggest the contribution that spinal stenosis (with or without spondylolisthesis, and spondylolysis with or without structural stenosis) makes in the patient's pain, and correlated our findings with MRI and positional X rays as well as with clinical outcomes. This is a third application of functional EMG that we have found quite useful clinically. It is possible that in herniated nucleus pulposus, this same extension might actually shorten the H reflex as a McKenzie-type maneuver. We have seen a few cases in which this mechanism seems likely, but have not studied it enough for inclusion here.

We are now ready to go over these three examples of functional EMG in detail. First, we will describe the methods we have found most useful in neurological thoracic outlet syndrome. Then we will devote a chapter to outlining the clinical confirmation of the methods' utility, along with drawbacks and unanswered questions. Following this, the next chapter will describe the way we perform the FAIR test for piriformis syndrome, and following that, a chapter will outline the clinical utility of functional EMG in clinical practice. The next chapter after that, Chapter 8, will deal with spinal stenosis and foraminal narrowing the same way: first we will describe what we do, then support its clinical value. In Chapter 9, we attempt to illustrate the usefulness of these functional tests with clinical case studies. Finally, in Chapter 10, we will sketch out other ways of using dynamic EMG in different clinical encounters and ways for the electromyographer to extend the methods presented in this book beyond the limits of what we have currently experienced.

References

1. Fishman, LM, Dombi, GW, Michaelsen, C, Ringel, S, Rozbruch, J, Rosner, B, Weber, C. "Piriformis syndrome: diagnosis, treatment, and outcome – a 10-year study." *Arch Phys Med Rehabil.* 2002 Mar;83(3):295–301.
2. Peng, PW, Tumber, PS. "Ultrasound-guided interventional procedures for patients with chronic pelvic pain – a description of techniques and review of literature." *Pain Physician.* 2008 Mar–Apr;11(2):215–24.
3. Betts, A. "Combined fluoroscopic and nerve stimulator technique for injection of the piriformis muscle." *Pain Physician.* 2004 Apr;7(2):279–81.
4. Lang, AM. "Botulinum toxin type B in piriformis syndrome." *Am J Phys Med Rehabil.* 2004 Mar;83(3):198–202.
5. Fishman, LM, Konnoth, C, Rozner, B. "Botulinum neurotoxin type B and physical therapy in the treatment of piriformis syndrome: a dose-finding study." *Am J Phys Med Rehabil.* 2004 Jan;83(1):42–50.
6. Childers, MK, Wilson, DJ, Gnatz, SM, Conway, RR, Sherman, AK. "Botulinum toxin type A use in piriformis muscle syndrome: a pilot study." *Am J Phys Med Rehabil.* 2002 Oct;81(10):751–9.

7. Fanucci, E, Masala, S, Sodani, G, Varrucciu, V, Romagnoli, A, Squillaci, E, Simonetti, G. "CT-guided injection of botulinic toxin for percutaneous therapy of piriformis muscle syndrome with preliminary MRI results about denervative process." *Eur Radiol.* 2001;11(12):2543–48, Epub 2001 May 12.
8. Rodrigue, T, Hardy, RW. "Diagnosis and treatment of piriformis syndrome." *Neurosurg Clin N Am.* 2001 Apr;12(2):311–9.
9. Foster, MR. "Piriformis syndrome." *Orthopedics.* 2002 Aug;25(8):821–5.
10. Indrekvam, K, Sudmann, E. "Piriformis muscle syndrome in 19 patients treated by tenotomy– a 1- to 16-year follow-up study." *Int Orthop.* 2002;26(2):101–3.
11. Fishman, LM, Anderson, C, Rosner, B. "BOTOX and physical therapy in the treatment of piriformis syndrome." *Am J Phys Med Rehabil.* 2002 Dec;81(12):936–42.
12. Chang, CW, Shieh, SF, Li, CM, Wu, WT, Chang, KF. "Measurement of motor nerve conduction velocity of the sciatic nerve in patients with piriformis syndrome: a magnetic stimulation study." *Arch Phys Med Rehabil.* 2006 Oct;87(10):1371–5.
13. Filler, AG, Haynes, J, Jordan, SE et al. "Sciatica of nondisc origin and piriformis syndrome: diagnosis by magnetic resonance neurography and interventional magnetic resonance imaging with outcome study of resulting treatment." *J Neurosurg Spine.* 2005 Feb;2(2)99–115.
14. Filler, AG. "Piriformis and related entrapment syndromes: diagnosis & management." *Neurosurg Clin N Am.* 2008 Oct;19(4):609–22.
15. Fishman, LM, Ardman, CA. *Cure Back Pain with Yoga.* W.W. Norton and Co., New York, June 2006.
16. Fishman, LM, Ardman, CA. *Sciatica: Diagnosis, Prevention and Cure of Spinal and Piriformis Problems.* W. W. Norton and Company, New York, November 2006.
17. Fishman, LM, Schaefer, MP:. "The piriformis syndrome is underdiagnosd." *Muscle Nerve.* November 2003;28(5):646–9.
18. Fritz, JM, Erhard, RE, Delitto, A, Welch, WC, Nowakowski, PE. "Preliminary results of the use of a two-stage treadmill test as a clinical diagnostic tool in the differential diagnosis of lumbar spinal stenosis." *J Spinal Disord.* 1997 Oct;10(5):410–6.
19. Whitman, JM, Flynn, TW, Childs, JD, Wainner, RS, Gill, HE, Ryder, MG, Garber, MB, Bennett, AC, Fritz, JM. "A comparison between two physical therapy treatment programs for patients with lumbar spinal stenosis: a randomized clinical trial." *Spine.* 2007 April 1;32(7):833–4.
20. Fritz, J. "A nonsurgical treatment approach for patients with lumbar spinal stenosis." *Phys Ther.* 9 Sept 1997;Vol 77 Number:964.
21. Sortland, O et al. "Functional myelograpy with metrizamide in the diagnosis of lumbar spinal stenosis." *Acta Radiol.* 1977;355(suppl):42–54.

Chapter 4
Neurological Thoracic Outlet Syndrome: Approaching a Pathognomonic Sign

Abstract It is ironic that in substantiating a diagnosis of exclusion such as thoracic outlet syndrome, it is critical to exclude an especially wide variety of other diagnoses. We first pare off vascular thoracic outlet syndrome, and make many exclusionary provisions before confirming that a functional electrodiagnostic test is positive with a fair-sized group of qualifying patients with impressive pain that bears no other ready explanation.

Keywords Paraesthesias · PML · Erb's point · Scalenus anticus · Scalenus medius · Vascular thoracic outlet syndrome · Clavicle · Coracoid process · Axillary nerve · Radial nerve · Musculoskeletal nerve · Ulnar nerve

Functional Identification of Thoracic Outlet Syndrome

Neurological thoracic outlet syndrome (NTOS), an entrapment syndrome, is a painful and debilitating neuromuscular condition that can neither be diagnosed by imaging studies nor, according to most researchers, by conventional EMG [1–3]. In many of the alleged cases of NTOS, also known as scalenus anterior syndrome and costoclavicular syndrome, there is no structural abnormality to be pictured, and if there is, its role as a pain generator is often open to question. Although there is hardly unanimity in the studies, most authors do agree that there is no reliable nerve conduction defect in the anatomical position of the standard electromyographic examination. Furthermore, the outcomes of both surgical and conservative treatment are controversial. The absence of a pathognomonic set of symptoms, the impression of multiple and elusive causation, disagreement about (and therefore absence of) any standard test for it, and less-than-impressive treatment combine to put NTOS on shaky ground and render it a diagnosis of exclusion.

In epidemiological terms, NTOS accounts for a widely variable percentage of upper extremity and shoulder pain [4, 5]. It has been estimated that 90% of the cases of thoracic outlet syndrome are neurological and that therefore NTOS is the most important of these clinical entities. But since diagnostic tests are variably understood

L.M. Fishman, A.N. Wilkins, *Functional Electromyography*,
DOI 10.1007/978-1-60761-020-5_4, © Springer Science+Business Media, LLC 2011

and evaluated, this information must be interpreted cautiously [6, 7]. We must go through the factors responsible for this uncertainty one by one:

Symptoms

Thoracic outlet syndrome is generally suggested by pain, paraesthesias, numbness, weakness and/or wasting of the upper extremity, especially in a distribution pattern corresponding to the divisions, cords or peripheral nerves, rather than a dermatomal or myotomal pattern, and especially if related to position.

These symptoms may also call to mind CVA, entrapments such as carpal tunnel syndrome, mononeuropathies, polyneuropathies and combinations of more than one radiculopathy, multiple sclerosis, cervical stenosis, and even Chiari-type and arteriovenous malformations. Each of these has, of course, legitimate and recognized means of diagnosis.

When considered at all, NTOS is generally admitted to the differential diagnosis for neurological symptoms in the arm and hand only after there are no longer reasons to suspect the more readily detectible axial conditions and appendicular conditions just mentioned.

Signs

Ironically, there is evidence in the literature favoring the idea that NTOS *should* be a diagnosis of exclusion. Nord et al. found that the false-positive rate of diagnosing NTOS by any of the usual tests was significantly higher in the presence of another diagnosis, carpal tunnel syndrome [8]. Adson maneuver (head turned to the ipsilateral side) and the Allen or Hallstead maneuver (head turned to the contralateral side), the costoclavicular maneuver, the elevated arm stress test, and supraclavicular pressure test were all falsely positive more than twice as frequently in the presence of carpal tunnel syndrome than they were when performed with normals. Such findings are particularly unnerving, so to say, given that most cases of thoracic outlet syndrome are supposed to involve the inferior trunk, the medial cord, or the ulnar nerve, and therefore the opposite side of the hand from median nerve entrapment at the carpal tunnel.

The suggestion is that these tests are actually more reliable when other diagnoses have been excluded! If valid, that paper vitiates the significance of all five of these diagnostic maneuvers unless other diagnoses have already been ruled out. Nevertheless, it offers *no* evidence that NTOS cannot veridically coexist with carpal tunnel syndrome or other conditions and it is unlikely that any such evidence could be forthcoming [4].

Provocative examination maneuvers were assessed in 200 upper extremities of 100 volunteers to determine the prevalence of positive responses in a typical population. The Adson, costoclavicular, and hyperabduction maneuvers were assessed for vascular and neurologic responses. Fifteen (7.5%) extremities had a Tinel's sign. The vascular response was present in 27 (13.5%) extremities for the Adson maneuver, 94 (47%) for the costoclavicular maneuver, and 114 (57%) for the hyperabduction maneuver. A neurologic response was present in 4 (2%) extremities for the Adson maneuver, 20 (10%) for the costoclavicular maneuver, and 33 (16.5%) for the hyperabduction maneuver. The vascular response is more common than the neurologic response in the general population.

There are two versions of the hyperabduction maneuver and are as follows:

1. Monitoring the pulse or listening for a supraclavicular bruit, the examiner maximally abducts and extends the shoulder and elbow, respectively, ostensibly bending the neurovascular bundle 90°.
2. The examiner monitors the radial pulse while the patient ipsilaterally and maximally rotates the head, inhales, abducts 90°, and shrugs both shoulders

In both maneuvers, pulsatile changes constitute a positive test.

Other studies find Adson's maneuver useful for identifying NTOS [9]; still others find its presence or absence an important element in prognosing the extent of post-surgical recovery [10]. . Dynamic musculoskeletal ultrasound gives some evidence favoring position-related neurological compression.

Mechanisms of Causation

NTOS is ostensibly present when neurological symptoms are due to stretch or compression of the distal elements of the brachial plexus and proximal segments of the major nerves arising from them. As distinct from vascular thoracic outlet syndrome, no signs of arterial or venous compromise such as claudication or cyanosis or non-neurogenic swelling, respectively, need to be present in NTOS [5, 11–13]. . Naturally, both conditions can coexist, e.g., after clavicular fracture or with cervical rib [6, 14–16] ,and may be fused together in the differential diagnosis as "thoracic outlet syndrome" pure and not so simple. Still, it is only the neurological aspects that concern us here.

Most often, NTOS is thought to involve the lower trunk, due to the T1 root's origin below the level of the first rib, and its consequent hooking over the first rib as it leaves the thorax, passing between the scalenus anticus and medius as it does so [5, 13, 16–12]. . The narrow gap between the clavicle and the first rib is commonly noted as the point of compression for the subclavian artery and vein, and the cords of the brachial plexus [17]. This spot is also just in front of the Virchow-Troisier lymph nodes that collect metastatic cells from the thoracic duct, which drains the entire body except the right arm. Adsons maneuver was classically intended to detect thoracic metastases as well as Pancoast tumors through subclavian arterial compression at this point.

In the age of MRI, NTOS is sometimes linked to excessive tone of the scalenus and/or omohyoid muscles (as Adson himself did at times) [5, 11, 15, 5] which exert pressure directly on the trunks, divisions, cords, or proximal nerves of the upper extremity, and which in turn may constrain the free movement of any element of the brachial plexus at the scalenii, omohyoid or pectoralis muscles, the first or cervical

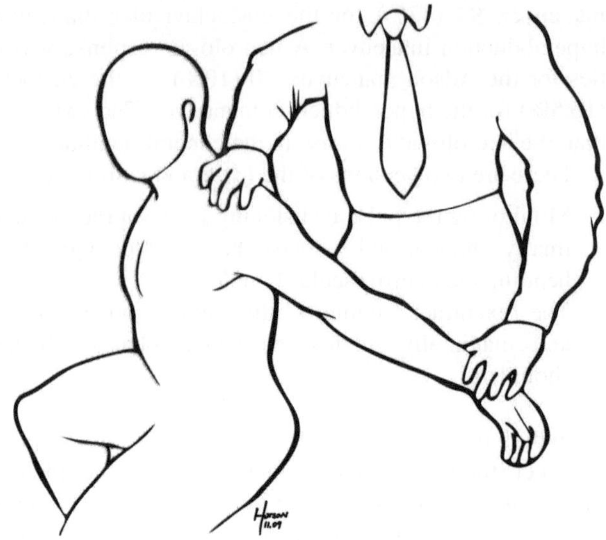

Fig. 4.1 Scalene maneuver: Monitoring the radial pulse, the examiner extends the shoulder and elbow as the patient ipsilaterally rotates and extends the neck and thoracic vertebrae, puffing out the chest. Diminution or disappearance of the pulse constitutes a positive test

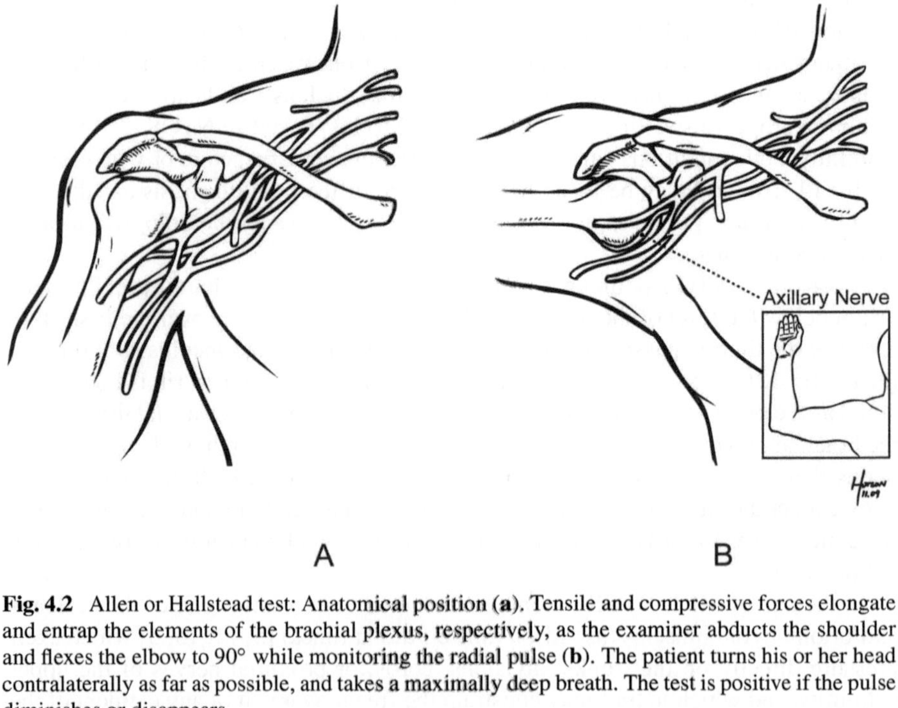

Fig. 4.2 Allen or Hallstead test: Anatomical position (**a**). Tensile and compressive forces elongate and entrap the elements of the brachial plexus, respectively, as the examiner abducts the shoulder and flexes the elbow to 90° while monitoring the radial pulse (**b**). The patient turns his or her head contralaterally as far as possible, and takes a maximally deep breath. The test is positive if the pulse diminishes or disappears

rib, the humeral head, the coracoid process, or elsewhere. Possible consequences include pain, paraesthesias, numbness, and occasionally weakness and ulnar wasting [16]. The symptoms are frequently heightened by abduction and/or flexion beyond 120° [5, 6, 14]. see Figs. 4.1, 4.2, and 4.3.

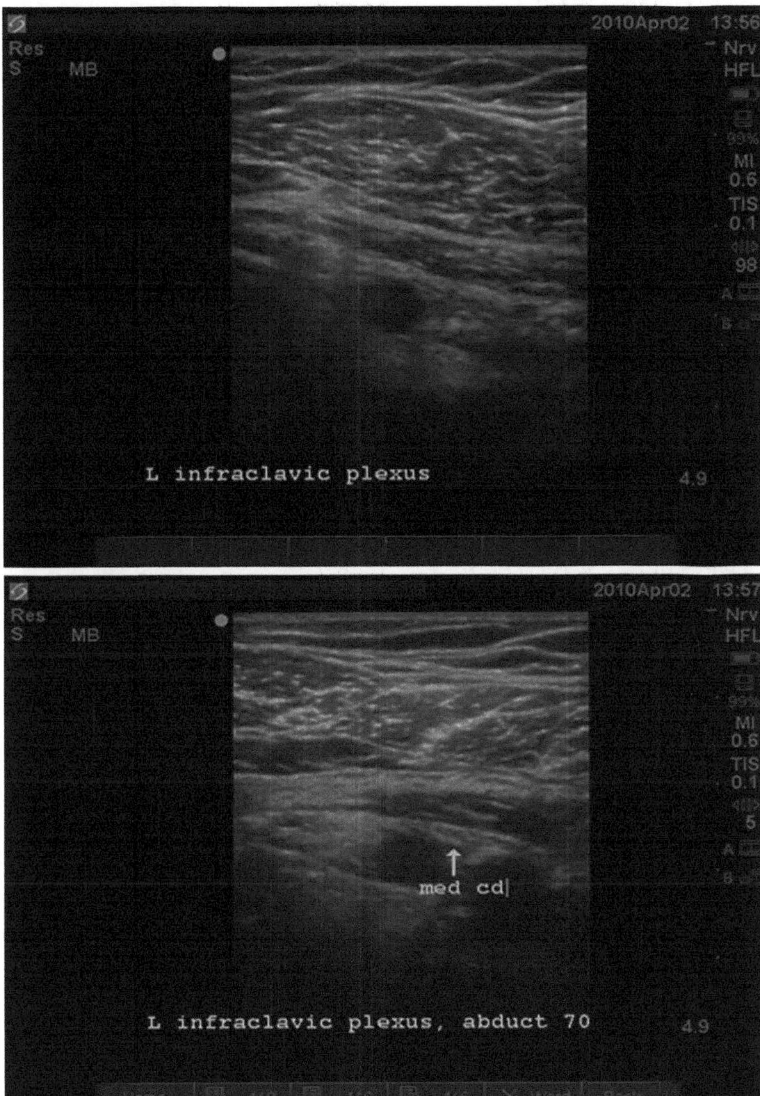

Fig. 4.3 Progressive abduction appears to cause neurological compression. The anatomical position gives no suggestion that there will be a scallop-shaped indentation of the posterior pectoralis by the radial nerve at 140° of abduction. Images courtesy of Benjamin M. Sucher, D.O., EMG Labs of AARA (Arizona Arthritis & Rheumatology Associates), Paradise Valley, AZ

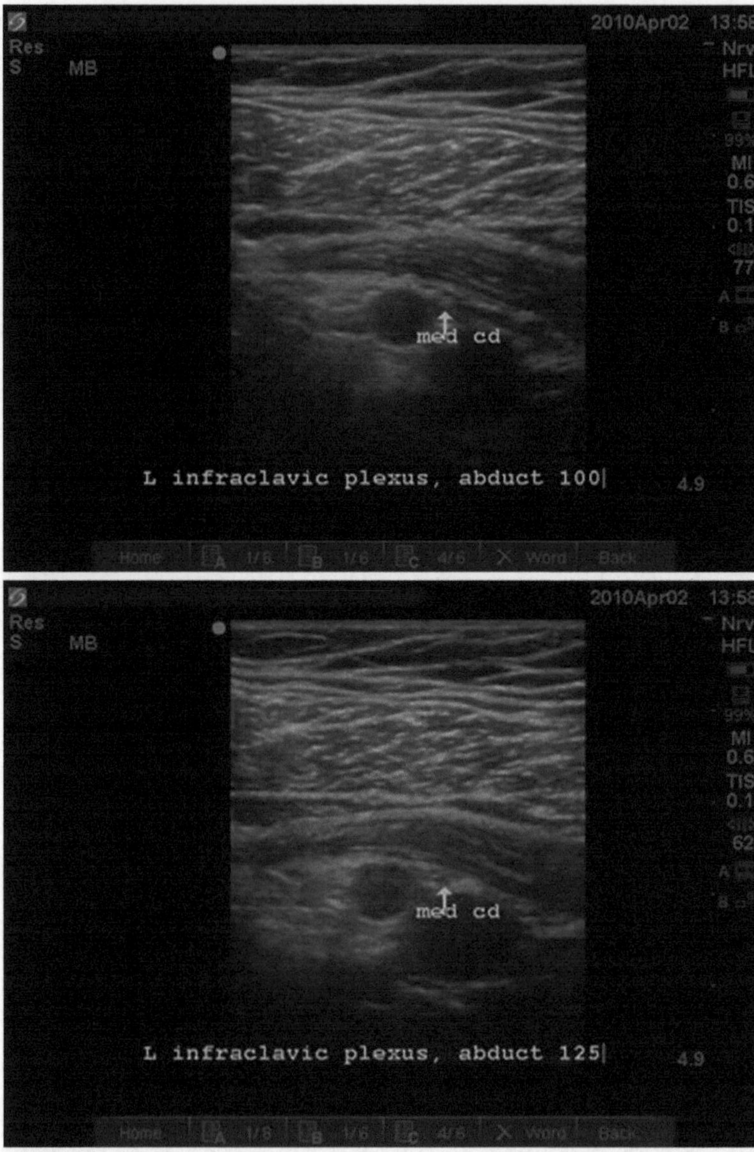

Fig. 4.3 (continued)

Other theories of the pathogenetic mechanism begin with poor posture [19, 20], a cervical rib [12–14] fibrous bands [5, 13–15], and other structures [14–5, 18, 20], overuse [19], and subtle but common anatomical variations such as penetration of the scalenii by nerve roots C5 and C6 [21].

In spite of, or perhaps because of this wealth of possible causes, NTOS, like the common cold, has been largely a diagnosis of exclusion [15, 22]. In part, this may be due to the ironic fact that these neurological symptoms have been diagnosed through one or another of the vascular tests we have just mentioned, and a cause of a manifestly functional condition is sought through MRI, a purely structural assessment.

Standard Test

Regardless of the cause, NTOS has been alternately alleged to and absolved from affecting sensory and motor nerve conduction, and in severe cases, causing nerve fiber disruption and damage [6, 14, 23]. Symptoms are often evinced by ipsilateral or contralateral head rotation (stiffening the scalenii, narrowing the distance between them, and stretching the omohyoid) [16, 5, 18], breathing deeply (raising the first rib) [5], and extreme flexion or abduction, coupled with external rotation of the arm in the coronal plane, maximally stretching (and thereby tightening) the roots, trunks, divisions, cords, and proximal nerves deriving from the brachial plexus, and increasing the pressure against them at key anatomical points [7, 14, 5]. Circumstances of contemporary living often seem to cause upper extremity pain in ways related to posture and position, i.e., functionally. Vigorous and repetitive activities such as continual lifting, practicing the serve in tennis, changing clothes, putting on seat belts, swimming, and other types of rhythmic upper extremity exertion may exacerbate the discomfort of NTOS as well, rendering the condition quite disabling [6, 19].

The plethora of opinions surrounding NTOS is due, in part, to lack of a definitive test for it [7]. Currently, MRI enables clinicians at least to form hypotheses based on soft tissue points of presumed contact identified pre-surgically. Can electrodiagnosis be of service here?

Electrophysiological evidence of NTOS has been sought, found, and disputed with equal zeal [1, 2]. Previous electrophysiological studies have focused on the ulnar nerve and the inferior trunk, with variable results [1, 2, 6]. Some studies have found EMG and NCV almost useless, except as a means of excluding other diagnoses [9] while others have seen useful confirmation of significant improvement with pre- and post-surgical comparisons [24]. Some have complained that the current studies only pick up gross injuries, suggesting that more sensitive techniques would be needed to detect conditions that are less severe [25]. Somatosensory-evoked potentials have also received mixed reviews from those who have worked with them in NTOS [25].

The questions have ranged from replicability, to means of measuring the distance from Erb's point across the axilla, and to methods of confirming a diagnosis so obtained [1, 2, 13]. This is the critical thing. If positive results from any test can be linked to successful specific treatment, surgical or otherwise, we are on the way to defining a viable clinical entity.

Treatment

When NTOS has been diagnosed, conservative treatment has been reasonably straightforward, but not dramatically effective, involving essentially restraint of extreme adduction and flexion during sleep [3] exercises that strengthen dorsal shoulder adductors [3, 5] ,postural training [3, 6, 5] ,and relieving trigger points in cervical muscles including the scalenii [18]. These methods have brought some patients significant relief [3, 4]. However, conservative means have been perceived as so uncertain that Sunderland actually gives criteria for their failure [26].

The number of surgical options has been inversely related to the certainty of their success, ranging from Adson's early excision of the scalenii and/or omohyoid [11, 14] to resection of the first rib [6, 12–14, 27–30] to thoracoplasty *via* various approaches [14, 20, 27–30]. Surgery for the condition has long been based on clinical diagnosis, failure of conservative treatment [26] and identification of a putative structural cause. For this as well as for other reasons, success rates have not always been high enough and post-operative complaints too common [6, 23, 27–30].

A New Test

Therefore, one may find enough motivation for considering new methods of diagnosis and treatment together. Somatosensory potentials were successful in a small trial (see Fig. 4.4). This chapter identifies patients with NTOS through prolongation of proximal motor latencies (PML) that appear in the Allen test (see Fig. 4.3). However, prolongation of PMLs will mean nothing unless its detection is coupled with successful treatment that is focused on the condition responsible for the patients' symptoms. Furthermore, progressive clinical improvement should correlate with reduced prolongation of the Allen test's PML in serial electrophysiological testing.

To review, Allen's maneuver has the patient abduct the affected arm 90°, externally rotate it 90°, revolve his or her head as far as practicable, and take the biggest possible breath. The rotation is contralateral. Allen test is positive if the radial pulse, generally taken at the wrist, is either significantly diminished or totally obliterated by these actions.

The mere presence of cervical ribs, whether unilateral or bilateral, does not necessarily mean that they are responsible for pains in the shoulder or arm. The factors responsible for reducing the length and the depth of the posterior cervical triangle determine whether or not pressure is produced on the subclavian artery and the brachial plexus. In some instances, when cervical ribs are absent, symptoms appear similar to those produced by their presence.
Alfred W. Adson [31]

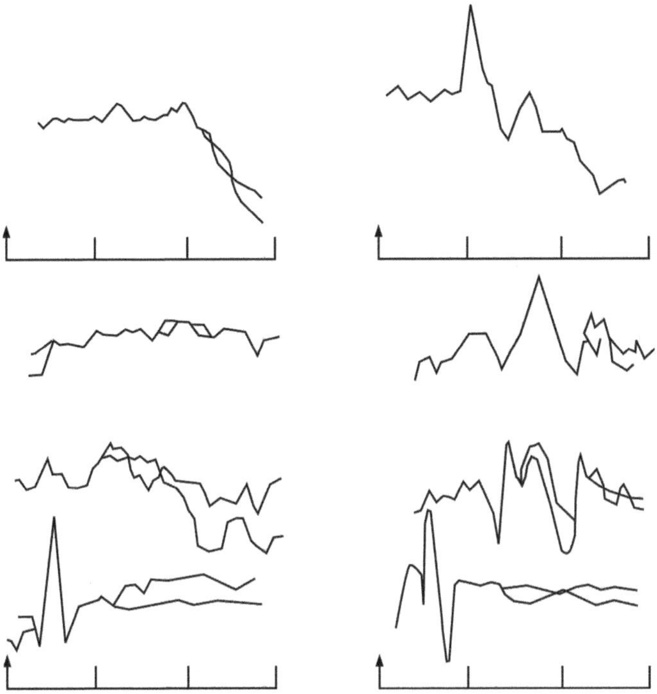

Fig. 4.4 Compare right (normal) SSEPs at somatosensory strip, cervical spine, and Erb's point with absent signals on *left*. At the elbow, *right* and *left* are comparable. This suggests compression between that location and the coracoid process. (ibid. pp. 278–80)

In the Clinical Context: Solving the Patient's Problem

The clinician's first job is to distinguish neurological thoracic outlet syndrome from its rarer relative, vascular thoracic outlet syndrome. Authors further differentiate arterial from venous types of vascular entrapment, considering cervical rib as a common cause of both, and pain as a common symptom. But subclavian arterial stenosis and aneurism are other arterial causes of ischemic symptoms, such as cyanosis and atrophy, while subclavian venous thrombosis may cause swelling and pain in the venous syndrome [9]. Although only ischemic pain and atrophy overlap with the painful numbness, paraesthesias and weakness that are typical of NTOS, confusion is almost inevitable, since, again, the provocative maneuvers all depend on a vascular sign. Still, NTOS has been estimated to comprise 90% of the cases of thoracic outlet syndrome [9].

We have had strong indications of NTOS using provocative maneuvers, with a possible dynamic anatomical explanation. Once the neurovascular bundle forms as the axillary artery crosses over its notch in the first rib, and joins the cords of the brachial plexus, the neurological and vascular structures travel together underneath the clavicle and out past the coracoid process, where they partially part ways. The provocative maneuvers stretch the elements that comprise the brachial plexus and approximate the structures that compress them, putting torsion especially on the axillary nerve, and pulling the axillary artery against the sharp edge of the first rib, and the undersides of both the clavicle and the arching hook of the coracoid process, while changing the angle of the scapula to which it is attached. Abduction also stretches the pectoralis muscle across the nerves' path.

So we know that there are vascular elements affected by a positive Allen's maneuver—that is what the test tests. We can reason that if the pulse vanishes, then the pressure on the brachial artery is equal to or greater than the systolic blood pressure. From a neurological point of view, if numbness, weakness, paraesthesias, or pain result quite quickly from the maneuver, then we might expect significant nerve compression. Although vascular compromise can indeed produce all of the above symptoms, minutes, not seconds, are necessary for any of them to show up in ischemia or reduced venous return.

From a neurological standpoint, a positive Allen maneuver must be added to a set of symptoms the timing of which can only be explained in terms of reversible nerve compromise. Thermal and spinning tests for semicircular canal dysfunction, blood pressure monitoring for orthostatic hypotension, straight leg raise, and even reflex testing meet this criterion. There must be a constant conjunction between the maneuver and the change in measurement or symptom. Structural factors that narrow neuroforamina with positional changes, such as turning the head, or, of course, a space-occupying entity such as a Pancoast tumor present the same timing too. It is not hard to see how NTOS got to be a diagnosis of exclusion.

But if pressure brought to bear by the Allen test almost immediately generates the patient's pain, paraesthesias, numbness, and possibly weakness, there ought to be some way to record and estimate its neurological effects. Something that would elevate NTOS from a diagnosis of exclusion to a diagnosis proper. We have found that there is reversible slowing of proximal motor nerve conductions and prolonged proximal motor latencies brought about by Allen's test.

The axillary nerve's circuitous course to the deltoid may make it sensitive to the Allen test. The Allen test may increase the intensity of contact between the scalenii and the brachial plexus, and raise its proximal motor latency (PML). Another possibility is that the fibers of the axillary nerve itself become entrapped more distally at the coracoid process or the pectoralis (see Figs. 4.1 and 4.2). Exactly where entrapment takes place, and whether individuals exhibiting axillary nerve PML prolongation would also have changes in conductions across the inferior trunk, medial cord, or ulnar nerve are subjects for further investigation. But we found fairly consistent rise in axillary PML with the Allen test in patients who appeared to have NTOS.

Grown Girl with Guitar

The first time we tried this was when a 28-year-old executive presented with 2 years of increasing pain, sensory changes, and weakness whenever she lifted her left arm to the frets of her guitar for more than a few seconds. She had had normal MRIs of the cervical spine and head, no problems on conventional EMG, and unremarkable X rays of the atlantooccipital junction and shoulder. Suspecting something functional, we asked her to bring in her guitar, and when she did, she could lay it in her lap and play without difficulty. When she raised it into the typical position, the pain and paraesthesias started almost immediately, and soon led to a mild/moderate sensory deficit at the left lateral upper arm. There was a decrease in the strength of abduction from 5−/5 to 4−/5 within a minute, and it lasted no more than half that after she brought the arm and the guitar down.

We gauged exactly how high she had to hold her hand on the neck of her guitar for the pain to begin, and found that Allen's test became positive right there, using the radial artery at the wrist. We found normal PML of 3.6 for axillary conductions from Erb's point to the deltoid, but it was replicably prolonged to 5.1 ms when we repeated the study in Allen's maneuver. The compound muscle action potential dropped from normal by 20% (needle electrode). Conductions to the teres minor were also prolonged from normal by the same maneuver, but only by 0.7 ms, and with no appreciable conduction block. Other conductions along the radial, musculocutaneous, and suprascapular nerves from Erb's point to the teres minor, triceps, biceps, and supraspinatus had normal PMLs in the anatomical position and did not change appreciably with the Allen maneuver. The same unchanging normalcy was seen with median and ulnar F waves, and in contralateral conventional and provocative axillary nerve studies.

EMG found a few positive sharp waves and polyphasia in the deltoid only.

We concluded that the young lady had a position-dependent NTOS, and treated her at first with myofascial work at the scalenii, scapular kinetics, and a figure-of-eight brace to reduce the distance that the nerve fibers had to travel from the neuroforamina to the deltoid muscle. She improved approximately 40–50% over the next month but went no further. She could now play one or two songs before the symptoms started.

We went to the next level then, and since it fit into an IRB-approved protocol we had for another project, injected her scalenus anticus and scalenus medius each with 2,500 Units of botulinum neurotoxin type B.

Within 6 days she was symptom-free, sitting for more than an hour-and-a-half with her guitar, prompting us to revise our IRB submission and seek to understand and replicate what had just happened. In botulinum neurotoxin injection, we had found a specific treatment that would validate or disprove the connection between neurological changes in the Allen test and neurological thoracic outlet syndrome. We applied for another IRB approval.

We restricted our study to patients who met the following three conditions:

1. Pain, paraesthesias, sensory deficit or weakness in the shoulder, upper arm, forearm, wrist or hand.
2. Disappearance of the radial or ulnar pulse at the wrist with Allen's maneuver: 90° abduction and 90° external rotation of the arm, and maximal contralateral or ipsilateral rotation of the head with maximal inhalation [14].
3. MRI ruling out cervical radiculopathy and EMG without evidence of paraspinal denervation, polyneuropathy, or other entrapment.

Since we aimed to show that these patients had NTOS, we were in the paradoxical position of excluding other diagnoses in the process of proving that NTOS was not a diagnosis of exclusion.

We used only Allen's maneuver, always comparing PML and (rarely) F wave in the anatomical position with PML or F wave in Allen's maneuver. We often made the comparison in more than one nerve, but determined which nerves to test by the physical examination. For example, if the dorsal forearm had positional paraesthesias and numbness, with weakness of finger and wrist extensors in more than 150° of flexion, we tested radial nerve conductions to the extensor indicis proprius.

Confirmation of the provocative electrophysiological test as a valid indicator of NTOS required a prolongation of the PML by Allen's maneuver ≥1.0 ms, 2 standard deviations beyond the upper value of normal for that conduction [32, 33].

We considered that abduction and external rotation of the humerus lengthen the linear path that upper extremity nerves must traverse to descend down the arm. This intensifies the pressure that the thoracic outlet muscles, the scalenii, pectoralis and omohyoid, exert on the trunks, divisions, and cords of the brachial plexus as they pass between these muscles. The position also increases the tensile strain on the cords and proximal nerves of the brachial plexus and the pressure the clavicle and the coracoid process exert on them.

Because of this, we took significant delay of M waves evoked through this positioning to be pathognomonic for NTOS. We reasoned that in some cases of NTOS, as the degree of external rotation in Adson's maneuver, the independent variable, is increased, the delay of the M wave, the dependent variable, would also increase (see Figs. 4.5 and 4.6).

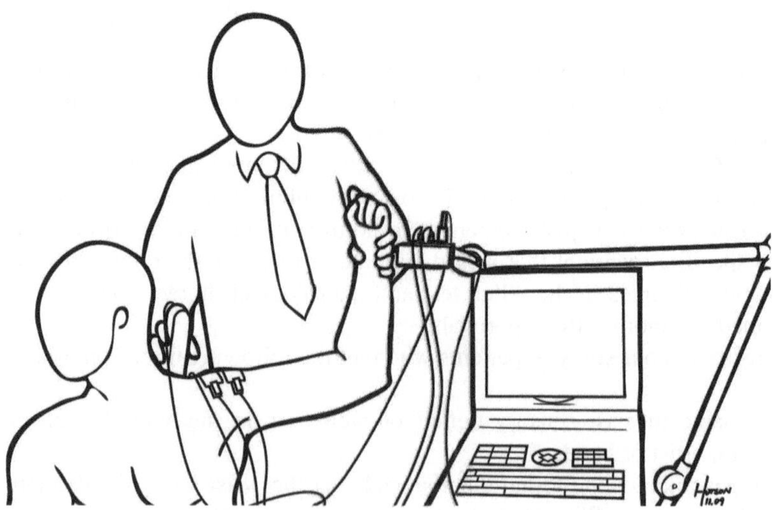

Fig. 4.5 Electrophysiological version of the Allen test

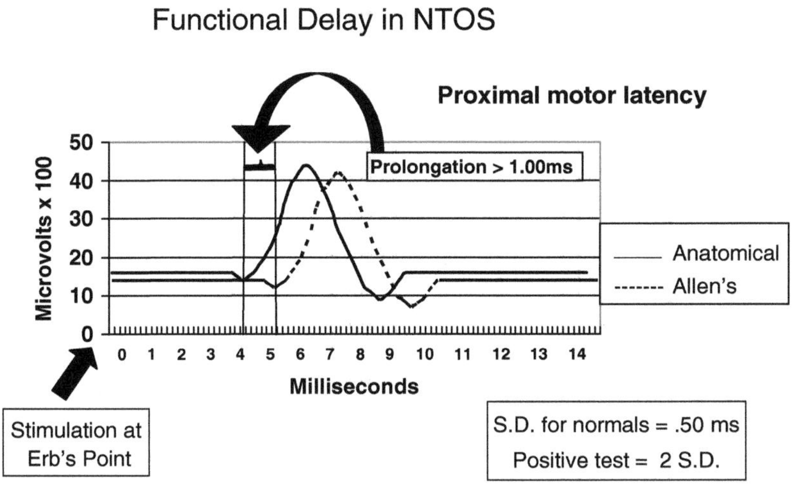

Fig. 4.6 NTOS was diagnosed when proximal motor latency from Erb's point to any muscle, obtained in the anatomical position, was prolonged by 1 ms (2 SD) or more by the Allen test. This standard deviation (.5 ms) represents conductions from Erb's point to proximal arm and dorsal thoracic muscles in normal subjects [31].

Since we were trying to validate this provocative test, we needed to isolate it from allied conditions. Hence there were extensive exclusionary criteria, as follows:

Cervical rib or anomalous tendinous band
Focal vascular disease (moderate atherosclerosis was acceptable)
Pregnant/nursing mother
Less than 18 years of age
Thrombocytopenia
Anticoagulation
Autoimmune disease

Allergy to or previous exposure to Bt-B, including previous history of botulism.

Cervical or ipsilateral shoulder, breast or pulmonary surgery
Neuromuscular disease
Weight below 106 pounds
Spastic torticollis or cervical dystonia
Vascular anomalies such as cervical steal syndrome
The protocol was approved by the IRB at Sound Shore Hospital, New Rochelle, New York.

We announced the study and request for patients on a New York radio station for 2 weeks, and soon had a fair number to examine and test. We used the anatomical distribution of the individual patient's motor and sensory symptoms to determine which nerves we would test. In overlapping cases, we would test all implicated nerves. For example, if medial and lateral volar areas had sensory deficits, we would look for distal motor latency differences in Allen's maneuver for the median and ulnar nerves.

We did not use F waves because of their inherent variability, and the likelihood that retaining the affected limb in the Allen test position for very long would affect the results, and possibly injure the patient. We felt it was reasonable that if 2 standard deviations' variation between two healthy limbs was significant, that such variation within the same limb in different positions would also be significant.

Making no claim to detect every case of NTOS, we found 33 patients who met the inclusion criteria within the initial 45 patients who eluded the exclusion criteria, and had sufficient prolongation of their proximal and in a few cases distal motor latencies. We could look for false positives, but not false negatives, since there are no really accepted criteria for NTOS. That of course is the point. Thirty of the patients were willing to undergo the full course of diagnosis and treatment.

The breakdown involves a number of different nerves, and both proximal motor latencies and F-waves. They are listed in Table 4.1. Although the axillary nerve was the most commonly found prolonged in this functional test, this cannot be taken to imply that it is the most, nor the most frequently affected in a clinically significant manner. It may only reflect that the axillary nerve was the most responsive to the Allen test.

All values were replicated by waiting 1–3 min and repeating the maneuver. It was unfortunate, but there was no satisfactory way to measure either the force applied, since it was often applied both at the elbow and the wrist, or the true angle, due to the mobility of the scapula. The provocative maneuver was sometimes mildly painful because we attempted to obtain a maximum delay that was consistent with patient well-being. Neither injuries nor protracted discomfort were seen. Both the maneuver and the stimulus applied at the brachial plexus were unpleasant, but many patients were openly grateful that someone had taken additional steps to find the cause of their complaints.

Once we had identified a unique characteristic that these patients shared—reversible delay of PML or F wave by the Allen test—the next step was to determine whether that characteristic could be linked to a successful treatment of their complaints. If so, we would have a cluster of symptoms, a definite test, and a method to address the condition detected by a positive test result. This might lift NTOS from the purgatory of "diagnosis of exclusion," confirm the value of a new technique based on dynamic nerve conduction changes, and simultaneously also validate the injection-plus-physical-therapy the patients received. We must turn to the conservative treatment most of these patients received and compare their outcomes with the subgroup of controls.

Table 4.1 The average PML delay induced by the Allen test was more than 3 standard deviations (SD) beyond the mean found in normals; the SD of that delay was quite close to the SD of PML in the anatomical position

Patient	Delay	Anatomical	Allen test	Comment
Axillary nerve				
1	2.3	3.7	6.0	
2	1.5	4.2	5.7	Lupus
3	1.3	4.1	5.4	
3	2.3	4.5	7.8	Lupus
4	1.1	5.5	6.6	Health club devotee
5	2.2	4.1	6.3	Weakness with abduction
6	1.8	4.3	6.1	
7	1.4	3.8	5.2	
8	1.8	4.7	6.5	
9	1.6	5.9	7.5	Football injury
10	0.4	4.4	4.8	
11	1.66	4.9	6.56	Morbid obesity
Radial nerve				
12	1.1	1.9	3.0	Snapping scaoula
13	1.7	3.1	4.8	63 yr. old skier
14	2.3	3.6	5.3	Fall
15	2.9	3.8	6.7	
16	1.4	26.9	28.3	F wave
17	1.6	12.0	13.6	S/P mastectomy
18	2.2	2.4	5.6	
Musculocutaneous				
19	1.8	3.7	5.5	severe shoulder pain
20	1.5	5.4	6.9	Fall
21	2.3	4.2	6.5	
22	0.6	4.4	5.0	
Ulnar				
23	1.9	23.1	25.0	F-wave, sensory loss and weakness
24	1.7	28.3	30	
25	2.1	27.5	29.6	F-wave
Suprascapular				
26	1.9	7.7	9.6	
27	2.5	7.0	9.1	Paraesthesias and sensory deficit
Median				
28	1.4	26.1	27.6	F-wave
29	1.4	27.7	29.1	
Thoracodorsal				
30	2.3	3.8	6.1	
Average delay	1.731			
Standard deviation	0.543			

References

1. Wilbourne, AJ, Lederman, RJ. "Evidence for conduction delay in thoracic-outlet syndrome is challenged." *N Engl J Med.* 1996;310:1052.
2. Smith, T, Trojaborg, W. "Diagnosis of thoracic outlet syndrome. Value of sensory and motor conduction studies and quantitative electromyography." *Arch Neurol.* 1987;44:1161.
3. Peet, RM, Hendrickson, JD, Gunderson, TP, Martin, GM. "Thoracic outlet syndrome: evaluation of a therapeutic exercise program." *Proc Mayo Clin.* 1956;31:265.
4. Rayan, GM, Jensen, C. "Thoracic outlet syndrome: provocative examination maneuvers in a typical population." *J Shoulder Elbow Surg.* 1995 Mar–Apr;4(2):113–17.
5. Travell, JG, Simons, DG. *Myofascial Pain and Dysfunction the Trigger Point Manual Volume 1.* Williams and Wilkins, Baltimore, 1983, p. 357.
6. Dawson, DM, Hallett, M, Millender, LH. *Entrapment Neuropathies.* 2nd Ed. Little Brown and Company, Boston/Toronto, 1990.
7. Plewa, MC, Delinger, M. "The false-positive rate of thoracic outlet syndrome shoulder maneuvers in healthy subjects." *Acad Emerg Med.* 1998 Apr;5(4):337–42.
8. Nord, KM, Kapoor, P, Fisher, J, Thomas, G, Sundaram, A, Scott, K, Kothari, MJ. "False positive rate of thoracic outlet syndrome diagnostic maneuvers." *Electromyogr Clin Neurophysiol.* 2008 Mar;48(2):67–74.
9. Sanders, RJ, Hammond, SL, Rao, NM. "Diagnosis of thoracic outlet syndrome." *J Vasc Surg.* 2007 Sep;46(3):601–4.
10. Ghoussoub, K, Tabet, G, Faraj, C, Sleilaty, G, Roukoz, S, Jebara, V. "Predictive factors of long-term functional rehabilitation in thoracic outlet syndromes: 85 patients." *Ann Readapt Med Phys.* Epub 2006 Apr;50(3):134–9, Dec 22. [Article in French].
11. Hood, DB, Kuehne, J, Yellin, AE, Weaver, FA. "Vascular complications of thoracic outlet syndrome." *Am Surg.* 1997 Oct;63(10):913–17.
12. Mayfield, FH. "Neural and vascular compression syndromes of the shoulder girdle and arms." In Vinken, PJ, Bruyn, GW (eds.). *Textbook of Clinical Neurology.* Vol. 7. American Elsevier, New York, 1976.
13. Hamlin, H, Pecora, D. "Subclavian segmental resection of the first rib for correction of subjacent neurovascular compression." *Am J Surg.* 1969;117:754.
14. Adson, AW. "Cervical ribs: Symptoms, differential diagnosis and indications for section of the insertion of the scalenus anticus muscle." *J Int College Surg.* 1951;16:546–59.
15. Roos, DB. "Congenital anomalies associated with thoracic outlet syndrome." *Am J Surg.* 1976;132:771.
16. Naffziger, HC, Brant, WT. "Neuritis of the brachial plexus mechanical in origin. The scalenus syndrome." *Surgic Gynecol Obstet.* 1938;67:722–30.
17. Ger, R, Abrams, P, Olson, TR. *Essentials of Clinical Anatomy.* 2nd Ed. Parthenon, New York and London, 2001, pp. 248–9.
18. Lon, C. "Myofascial pain syndromes: part 2- syndromes of the head, neck and shoulder girdle." *Henry Ford Hospital Med Bull.* 1956;4:22–8, Quoted in Travell, JG, Simons, DG. *Myofascial Pain and Dysfunction the Trigger Point Manual Volume 1.* Williams and Wilkins, Baltimore, 1983.
19. Frankel, SA, Hirata, I, Jr. "The scalenus anticus syndrome and competitive swimming." *JAMA.* 1971;215:1796–8.
20. Wilbourn, JA, Porter, JA. "Thoracic outlet syndrome." *Spine.* 1988;2:57.
21. Grant, JCB. *An Atlas of Human Anatomy.* 7th Ed. Williams and Wilkins, Baltimore, 1978, Figs. 9-46 and 9-83.
22. Franklin, GM, Fulton-Kehoe, D, Bradley, C, Smith-Weller, T. "Outcome of surgery for thoracic outlet syndrome in Washington state workers′ compensation." *Neurology.* 2000 Nov 28;55(10):1594–5.
23. Ersche, HC, Razzuk, MA. "Management of the thoracic outlet syndrome." *N Engl J Med.* 1972;286:1140.

24. Han, S, Yildirim, E, Dural, K, Ozisik, K, Yazkan, R, Sakinci, U. "Transaxillary approach in thoracic outlet syndrome: the importance of resection of the first-rib." *Eur J Cardiothoracic Surg.* 2003 Sep;24(3):428–33.
25. Yainnikas, C. In Chiappa, KH *Evoked Potentias in Clinical Medicine.* Raven Press, New York, 1989, pp. 278–280.
26. Sunderland, D. *Nerves and Nerve Injuries.* 2nd Ed. Churchill Livingstone, London, 1978.
27. Cherington, M, Happer, I, Mechanic, B, Parry, L. "Surgery for thoracic outlet syndrome may be hazardous to your health." *Muscle Nerve* 1986;9:632–4.
28. Bhattacharya, V, Hansrani, M, Wyat, MG, Lambert, D, Jones, NAG. "Outcome following Surgery for Thoracic Outlet Syndrome." *Eur J Vasc Endovasc Surg.* 2003 Aug;26(Issue 2):170–5.
29. Oates, SD, Daley, RA. "Thoracic outlet syndrome." *Hand Clin.* 1996 Nov;12(4):705–18.
30. Kline, DG, Judice, DJ. "Operative management of selected brachial plexus lesions." *J Neurosurg.* 1983;58:631–49.
31. Adson, AW. "Cervical ribs: the symptoms, differential diagnosis and indications for section of the insertions of." *J Int College Surg.* 1951 Nov;15(5):546–59.
32. Delisa, JA, Mackenzie, L, Baran, EM. *Manual of Nerve Conduction Velocity and Somatosensory Evoked Potentials.* 2nd Ed. Raven Press, New York, 1987.
33. Kimura, J. *Electrodiagnosis in Diseases of Nerve and Muscle: Principles and Practice.* 2nd Ed. F.A. Davis and Co., Philadelphia, 1999.

Chapter 5
Treating Neurological Thoracic Outlet Syndrome Identified by a Provoked Electromyographic Sign: Analysis of the Data

Abstract Having isolated a group of patients for whom a functional electrophysiological test is positive, we then treated the patients in a manner that would specifically address thoracic outlet syndrome. Direct injection of botulinum neurotoxin into the scalenus anticus and medius relieved pain and contemporaneously reduced the positivity of the test, suggesting that the functional maneuver is sensitive to the pathogenetic mechanism. After 6–8 weeks, as the botulinum toxin's efficacy waned, both pain and positivity of the functional maneuver increased somewhat. Fortunately, physical therapy kept both under some control.

Keywords Synaptobrevin · VAMP · Bt-B · Suprascapular · Thoracodorsal · Long thoracic · Radiculopathy · Cervical · Chemodenervation · Visual Analogue Scale (VAS) · Pathogenetic mechanism · Physical therapy · Injection

Treatment of Thoracic Outlet Syndrome Based on Dynamic Changes in Nerve Conduction

Finding a neurological correlate to a narrowly defined set of symptoms is interesting, but in itself, useless. To have value in clinical medicine, dynamic electrodiagnosis must have some bearing on patient outcome. We designed a treatment that would only affect neurological entrapment at the thoracic outlet, specific to the mechanism of NTOS. It would not be likely to have an effect on symptoms due to radiculopathies, neuropathies, nor other more distal entrapments.

The patients who satisfied the inclusion and exclusion criteria in Chapter 4 and replicably showed at least a two standard deviation prolongation of the normal values of proximal or distal motor latencies (PML or DML) or F-waves in an upper extremity nerve during the Allen test were taken to have neurological thoracic outlet syndrome (NTOS).

In an IRB-authorized study, they were divided into three groups. Patients were either controls or injected double blindly with 2,500 or 5,000 units botulinum neurotoxin type B (Bt-B) in scalenus anticus and medius muscles (Table 5.1).

L.M. Fishman, A.N. Wilkins, *Functional Electromyography*,
DOI 10.1007/978-1-60761-020-5_5,

Table 5.1 Control and intervention groups

Group	Number	Female	Age	Weight	Left
Control	9	5	52	144.4	7
2,500 U	10	4	48	155.5	7
5,000 U	10	7	46	138.3	8
Mean	29		49	146.1	

All the patients, regardless of their grouping, received identical physical therapy consisting of figure-of-eight bracing, myofascial release work and modalities at the scalenii, and postural training.

We followed the patients with serial PML or F-wave studies of prolongation in Allen's maneuver, visual analogue scale (VAS) ratings, and adverse-effects profiles at weeks 2, 4, 8, 10, and 12. The main outcome measures, then, were VAS, serial functional electrophysiological results, i.e., changes in the PML or F-wave in the Allen test, and measure of any adverse effects from the medicinal injections, the physical therapy, or the serial testing.

Summing up the data from Chapter 4, the patients' nerves that conducted more slowly in Allen's maneuver were mainly the axillary, musculocutaneous, and radial nerves. In this chapter, we will see that the mean improvement in VAS of patients receiving Bt-B injections in the scalenii was greater at 4, 8, and 12 weeks than the controls. ($p < 0.001$, 0.012, 0.033, respectively; overall $p = 0.004$). PML and F-wave delays during the Allen test decreased in all groups of patients over that time period, but significantly moreso in those receiving the Bt-B injections. The chief adverse effects of Bt-B, dry mouth and dysphagia, peaked at weeks 2–4, resolving by week 8, and are known effects of Bt-B, and not of the physical therapy nor the testing.

Getting well ahead of the story, it appeared that Bt-B injections with physical therapy were more effective than physical therapy alone in treating NTOS that was detected through the dynamic electrophysiological testing. Secondarily, scalenus anticus and medius tension seemed relevant to the pathogenesis of some NTOS. We must now look at this in detail.

The heart of this proof-of-concept investigation is injection of botulinum neurotoxin type B. It is this intervention that is really quite specific to the diagnosis of NTOS. Although it could be argued, perhaps plausibly, that a figure-of-eight brace, the physical therapy, and even the attention paid to these patients had other effects that account for their improvement, it is difficult to find a way in which Bt-B would alter a radiculopathic or other central condition, orthopedic difficulties at the shoulder, or more peripheral entrapments.

What Is Botulinum Neurotoxin Type B?

The seven serologically distinct botulinum toxins designated A through G share a common structural organization consisting of one heavy chain and one light chain polypeptide linked by a single disulfide bond [1]. These toxins inhibit acetylcholine release at the neuromuscular junction through a series of steps: After heavy-chain neurospecific binding and receptor-mediated endocytosis, the translocated light chain acts as a zinc-dependent protease inside the cell, cleaving synaptic-vesicle-associated membrane protein (VAMP or synaptobrevin), a substance critical to neurotransmitter exocytosis and release. The small vesicles of acetylcholine are trapped within the neuron, unable to leave, and are prevented from crossing the synaptic cleft of the myoneural junction to stimulate the muscle.

By inhibiting the release of neurotransmitter, Bt-B produces flaccid paralysis at the myoneural junction adjacent to the site of its injection [1, 2].. It is not recognized to produce any effect more distally on motor or sensory nerves. Apart from its few adverse effects, Bt-B has only local action. This was an important safety feature since the entire brachial plexus lies between the scalenus anticus and medius, and the phrenic nerve crosses medially in front of the scalenus anticus. But Bt-B will have effect only on myoneural junctions. In this respect, it is an extremely local treatment, only affecting nerve fibres terminating at the site of its injection.

Dosages of up to 25,000 units have been employed without changes in the clinical profile of side effects of Bt-B. In a study of 57 patients, at 20,000–25,000 units, all but nine of whom had previous exposure to botulinum toxin type A, Bt-B toxin was tolerated well enough to receive additional doses in each of the 57 patients. Groups of patients above and below 65 years of age have had similar adverse-effect profiles [3].

Clinical studies indicate that at doses of 5,000–10,000 units, the medication suppresses neurotransmission for 8–12 weeks [3]. Some researchers hold botulinum neurotoxin type A, Botox, to be approximately 50–60 times stronger than Bt-B, accounting for the larger doses used here. Otherwise botulinum neurotoxins A and B have very similar properties.

Injection

Qualifying patients were placed in the control group or double blinded and randomized with respect to dosage of Bt-B.

Non-control patients received scalenus anticus and scalenus medius injections of either 2,500 units or 5,000 units of Bt-B, given in two equal doses of 625 units or 1,250 units in each muscle. In bilateral cases, and cases in which more than one nerve was involved, the more or most severely affected side was chosen for injection, and that nerve, the nerve most significantly prolonged by the Allen maneuver, was studied serially. Examiners were careful not to change anything else such as needle depth or stimulus intensity while performing the Allen test, and thereby possibly alter nerve conduction velocity or its measurement [4].

Patients were injected at the proximal and distal ends of the middle third of the scalenus anticus and medius muscles, avoiding the most dangerous areas vis-à-vis the brachial plexus, the phrenic nerve, the jugular vein, the carotid artery, and the thoracic duct. The more superior injection in each muscle was approximately 1.5 in.

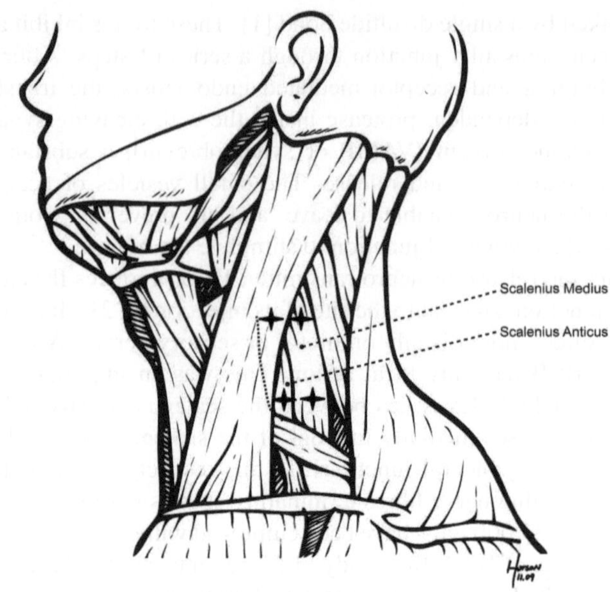

Fig. 5.1 The scalenus anticus and medius may be separated from the sternocleidomastoid by a deep breath and from the omohyoid through their orientation with ipsilateral and inferior head rotation. They originate from the anterior aspect of C2–C7 transverse processes, with the cervical nerve roots emerging, logically, between them. Injection is actually more difficult to the scalenus anticus than the medius due to the subclavian vein and phrenic nerve traversing the neck anterior to the anticus. The brachial plexus is quite low and since Bt-B is effective only at myoneural junctions, it is relatively uninvolved. The subclavian and axillary arteries, traveling with the plexus in a neurovascular bundle, are identified by their pulse [5]

inferior to the styloid process. The second was approximately 1.0–2.0 in. distal to the first (Fig. 5.1).

A 1.5-inch #25 teflon-coated injectable EMG needle was oriented horizontally, at a point giving good interference pattern on maximal contraction, to a depth of approximately 0.5 in. for each injection. Physical therapy and figure-of-eight bracing began within 1 week of injection.

Physical Therapy

The therapeutic regimen was designed to restore pain-free movement, relieve mechanical pressure at points of muscular and osseous contact, and correct postural abnormalities (kyphosis) that might have contributed to the severity of NTOS. The program had five stages, which were as follows:

1. Therapeutic use of 1.5 W/cm^2 ultrasound $\times$ 8–12 min and electrical stimulation at 80–150 Hz for 8–12 min on the scalenii.

2. Myofascial release involving affected tissue planes for 10–12 min.
3. Manual medical, muscle–energy, and strain–counterstrain techniques to restore lower cervical and scapular mobility.
4. Scalenus stretching exercises with postural/external compression work.
5. Appropriate standard bracing: a figure-of-eight brace worn at least 8 h during the day.

Therapy continued twice weekly for 12 weeks or until a patient was symptom-free for one full week, whichever occurred first. Further therapy was according to the agreement among the prescribing physician, physical therapist, and patient, but these further data are not analyzed here.

The protocol was distributed to each physical therapist treating control and intervention patients enrolled in the study, regardless of location. This description of physical therapy for NTOS was and still is available at www.sciatica.org.

Scheduled Follow-Up Visits

Subsequent visits were scheduled for weeks 2, 4, 8, 10, and 12. However, patient volition and clinical conditions actually spread these visits out over somewhat longer periods of time. Each patient encounter included the following:

Subjective: VAS rating [6].

Objective:

1. Repeat measure of PML or F-wave prolongation by Allen's maneuver.
2. Review of systems with specific attention to known adverse effects of Bt-B [7, 8] and anticipated adverse effects of the prescribed physical therapy and the repeated provocative maneuver.
3. The question: "Has anything happened since we saw you last that you think might be related to the injection of medication, the physical therapy, or the electrophysiological testing?"

Analysis of the Data

Age, weight, involved side, duration of symptoms, VAS pain ratings, adverse events, and Bt-B dosage were analyzed using paired two-tailed *t*-tests and analysis of covariance (ANCOVA).

Results

Thirty patients entered the study. A flare-up of systemic lupus erythematosis caused one patient drop out after week 2. Ten patients were included in the 2,500 unit and

Table 5.2 In nine patients more than one nerve showed significant delay (more than 1.0 ms) in Allen's maneuver*

Average age, weight, side, symptom duration, and nerve involvement*

Group	(n)	Age	Weight	Left	Yrs	Ax.	Musc.	Rad.	Med.	Ul.	Sup.	Tho.
Control	9	52	144.4	7	2.65	5	2	0	1	0	1	0
2,500 U	10	47.8	155.5	7	3.27	5	1	4	1	2	1	1
5,000 U	10	46.3	138.3	4	1.78	7	2	4	1	1	0	0
Mean	29	48.7	146.1		2.57							

Only the nerve showing the greatest delay at initial examination was followed to measure serial recovery, but all nerves with significant delay are tabulated here.
Yrs, years of symptoms; Ax., axillary; Musc., musculocutaneous; Rad., radial; Med., median; Ul., ulnar; Sup., suprascapular; Tho., thoracodorsal.

10 in the 5,000 unit arms of the study, with nine patients maintained as controls (Table 5.2).

Average age and weight for control and 2,500 unit and 5,000 unit groups were as follows: 49.4 years, 144.4 pounds; 47.8 years, 155.5 pounds; and 46.3 years, 138.3 pounds, respectively. Average duration of symptoms for the three groups was 2.7, 3.3, and 1.8 years, respectively, with the axillary nerve involved in 44% of cases, radial nerve in 20%, musculocutaneous nerve in 13%, and a small number of significant median, ulnar, suprascapular, and thoracodorsal nerve conductions slowing in Allen's maneuver (see Table 5.2).

Results of Scalenus Injections and Physical Therapy

Clinical recovery curves (VAS) suggested a significant beneficial effect following Bt-B injection at both dosages and physical therapy for all three groups, at weeks 4, 8, and 12, and overall ($p = 0.001$, 0.012, 0.033, and 0.004, respectively) (see Table 5.4 and Figs. 5.2, 5.3, 5.4, 5.5, and 5.6).

Patients' clinical courses strongly suggested that while physical therapy alone was effective, the injections of Bt-B sped that recovery along substantially. Further indication of the medicine's efficacy came from the unfortunate fact that the dramatic improvements experienced in the first weeks following its injection tended to diminish at the10th through 12th week, which approximates the length of time that Bt-B is effective in vitro. See Tables 5.3, 5.4, 5.5 and Figs. 5.2, 5.3, 5.4, 5.5, and 5.6.

The steep decline of the curve in the first 2 weeks is predicted by the 5–7 days of onset of Bt-B injection (Table 5.4).

Intervention group improvement was most dramatic at week 2, but greatest at week 6, when the average VAS score had dropped 57.2% overall, and 55.9 and 58.4% in the groups receiving 2,500 units and 5,000 units of Bt-B, respectively, versus 11.2% for the control group (see Table 5.3 and Figs. 5.2, 5.3, 5.4, 5.5, and 5.6).

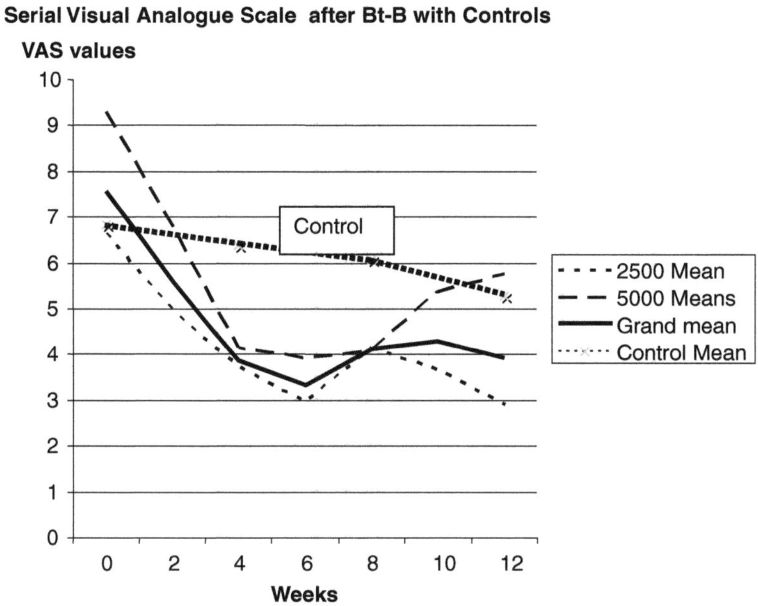

Fig. 5.2 Serial visual analogue scale values for intervention patients and controls. Patients receiving Bt-B 5,000 units averaged nearly two points higher at onset than those receiving Bt-B 2,500 units. Nevertheless their differences at 4–8 weeks were slight. Both groups improved significantly more than controls during the 3-month period in which Bt-B is effective

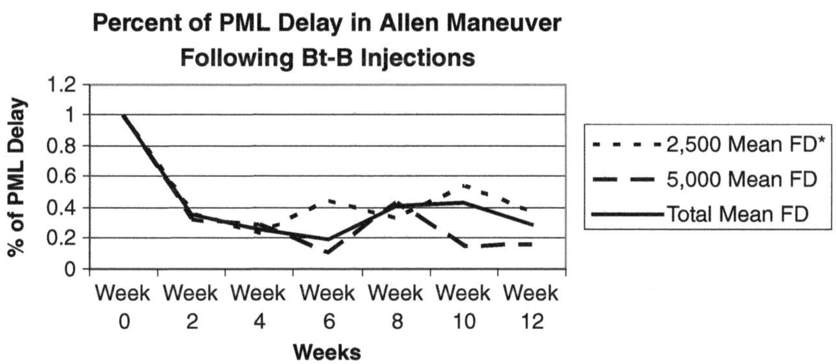

Fig. 5.3 Fractional reduction of proximal motor latency delay (Allen test – Anatomical) in conductions from Erb's point to deltoid or other muscle. Patients injected with Bt-B made faster and overall fuller clinical improvement than uninjected patients given the same regimen of physical therapy

Although their VAS and adverse-effect data were good, more than half the control group refused serial testing, and their electrophysiological data were too scanty to bear fruitful analysis.

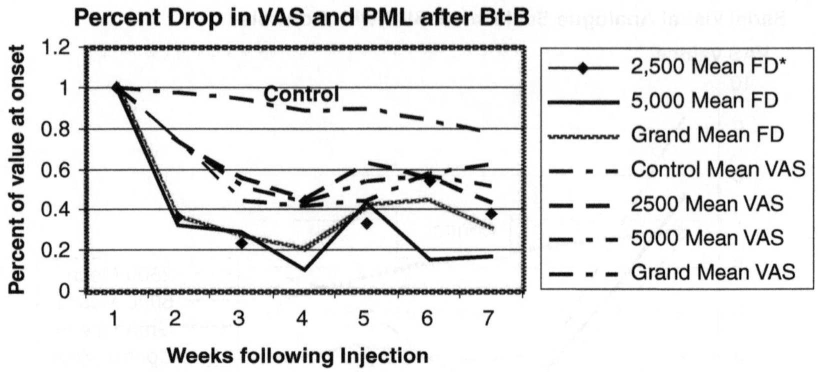

Fig. 5.4 The percent of initial pain on the VAS and percent of initial functional delay in the Allen test were similar

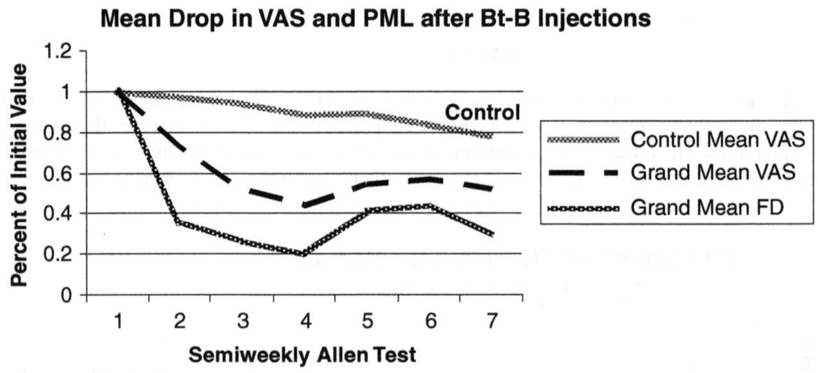

Fig. 5.5 The parallel variation of pain on the visual analogue scale and delay of proximal motor latency in the Allen test suggests we were measuring what hurt

Injected patients' PML and F-wave prolongation in Allen's maneuver was minimized in week 6 when it was reduced 55.6% in the 2,500-unit group, 89.7% in the 5,000-unit groups, and 72.7% overall. Considerable gains were retained over the 12-week study period (see Tables 5.3, 5.4, 5.5 and Figs. 5.2, 5.3, 5.4, 5.5, and 5.6).

It seemed evident that both the patients' symptoms and the electrophysiological evaluation of the Allen test—a provocative maneuver—were beneficially influenced by Bt-B injections. Patients receiving higher dosages of Bt-B delivered at the scalenus anticus and medius revealed a dose-related effect. This suggested that the injected medicine was effective, and as a corollary that the sites of its delivery are active in the pathogenesis of the condition.

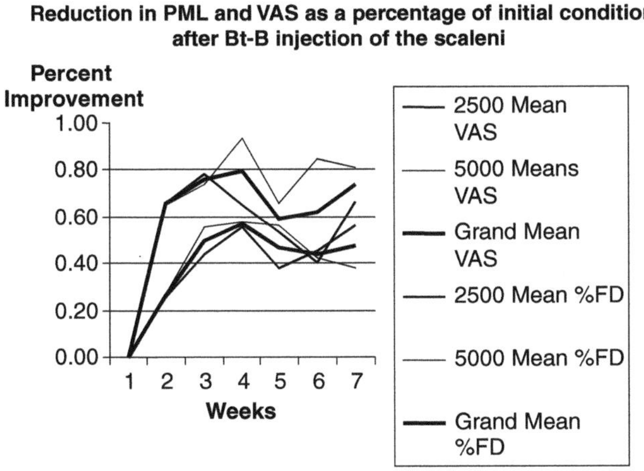

Fig. 5.6 Reduction in PML and VAS after Bt-B injection of the scalenii as a percentage of initial condition. Parallel decrease in pain and functional delay represented as percent reduction in functional delays and VAS after treatment by weeks. Proximal motor latency (PML) delays during the Allen test decreased substantially after scalenus injection of Bt-B and PT. This quite closely paralleled clinical improvement (VAS). This is perhaps the strongest suggestion that the functional delay brought about by the Allen test actually measures the symptom-producing pathology

Table 5.3 Serial reports on the visual analogue scale: controls and injected patients

Bi-weekly Visual Analogue Scale scores by group							
Group	0 week	2 weeks	4 weeks	6 weeks	8 weeks	10 weeks	12 weeks
Control mean	6.8	6.6	6.4	6.0	6.1	5.7	5.3
Std Dev	1.6	2.5	2.1	2.4	2.7	2.9	2.5
% Improvement		2.9	6.0	11.2	11.0	16.2	22.5
Mean: 2,500 unit	6.7	4.9	3.7	3.0	4.2	3.7	2.9
Std Dev	2.1	2.8	2.9	2.7	3.0	2.9	3.1
% Improvement		26.2	44.3	55.9	38.1	45.4	56.4
Mean: 5,000 unit	9.3	6.8	4.1	3.9	4.1	5.4	5.8
Std Dev	0.8	1.9	2.2	2.4	1.1	1.7	1.9
% Improvement		27.5	56.1	58.4	56.7	42.7	38.6
Grand mean	7.6	5.6	3.9	3.3	4.1	4.3	3.9
Std Dev	2.2	2.6	2.6	2.5	2.4	2.6	3.0
% Improvement of injected patients		26.5	49.0	56.1	45.7	43.4	48.5

Graphic representations suggested that the duration of the dramatic improvement coincided with the length of time for which Bt-B is active as well. See Figs. 5.2 and 5.3.

Of perhaps even greater interest to the electromyographer is that the courses were not merely contemporaneous, but nearly congruent as well. Greater improvement in

Table 5.4 Scalenus injection of botulinum neurotoxin type B with physical therapy was significantly more effective in relieving symptoms at the higher dose, and significantly more effective than physical therapy alone at both dosages

Assessment of Bt-B and physical therapy treatment for NTOS
VAS following Bt-B injection to patients with NTOS asdefined by 1.0 ms delay in Allen's maneuver

2,500 units	Mean	SE	N	5,000 units	Mean	SE		n
Week 4–week 0	–2.92	0.81	13		–5.14	0.89		7
Week 8–week 0	–2.5	0.93	10		–5.42	0.65		6
Week 12–week 0	–3.44	0.83	10		–3.75	0.87		6
Mean: week 0*	–2.53	0.54	10		–4.18	0.52		7
Controls	Mean	SE	N		Mean treated–mean control	SE	T	p-Value
Week 4–week 0	−0.44	0.28	9		−3.26	0.99	−3.29	0.001
Week 8–week 0	−0.78	0.5	9		−2.82	1.03	−2.74	0.012
Week 12–week 0	−1.56	0.5	9		−2	0.88	−2.27	0.033
Mean–week 0*	−0.93	0.4	9		−2.18	0.69	−3.15	0.004

*(Week 2 to week 12)–week 0.

Table 5.5 Fractional reduction of proximal motor latency delays in the Allen test: (subsequent values)/(initial values) after botulinum neurotoxin type B injections

Serial reduction in proximal motor latency delay in the Allen test after Bt-B injection in patients with NTOS as defined by 1 ms positional delay

Group/week	Week 0	Week 2	Week 4	Week 6	Week 8	Week 10	Week 12
2,500 mean %FD*	0	0.6349	0.7639	0.5556	0.6667	0.4583	0.625
5,000 mean % FD	0	0.6741	0.7129	0.8965	0.5654	0.8448	0.8344
Total mean %FD	0	0.6421	0.7393	0.809	0.5887	0.5691	0.7062

*%FD = reduction in functional delay of proximal motor latency in Allen's maneuver divided by proximal motor latency seen just prior in anatomical position.

VAS at a given date in the 3-month study period generally coincided with a reduced delay in proximal motor latency in the Allen test on that date (see Figs. 5.5 and 5.6).

Summing up the experiences and improvements of both measures, the clinical and the electrophysiological, in all three groups, the controls and those receiving injections of 2,500 units and 5,000 units of BT-B, the resulting profiles are strikingly parallel.

Because statistics cannot always be trusted to mean what they are alleged to mean, we analyzed the data from another point of view as well. Using the initial pre-treatment values as unity, we plotted the reduction in VAS versus the percentage difference in Allen-test delay over time (see Fig. 5.5).

Although the five-stage physical therapy might possibly, perhaps even plausibly, have beneficial effects in these patients for a number of reasons, the specificity of botulinum neurotoxins, acting at the neuromuscular junction and not elsewhere, again mitigates in favor of the important specific causative role of the scalenii in most of these cases of NTOS. These two measures vary together. Either one of them is causing the other, or there is some third thing that is causing both of them. This constant conjunction of their movement in serial studies over time gives some fundamental support to the idea that the functional electrodiagnostic evaluation of the Allen test, a provocative maneuver, is sensitive to the pathogenetic mechanism here (Fig. 5.6).

If the improvement we see in these patients reliably can be predicted for other people who show functional prolongation of PMLs and other measures of conduction velocity across the thoracic outlet, then at least some cases of NTOS may be diagnosed without the exclusion of any other diagnoses, let alone all.

Our purpose is to show the value of functional electromyographic studies; this is the first example. The second example has significantly more evidence to support it. We must now turn to piriformis syndrome and the FAIR test.

References

1. Simpson, LL. "The origin, structure, and pharmacological activity of botulinum neurotoxin." *Pharmocol Rev.* 1981;33:155–88.
2. Simpson, LL. "The actions of clostridial toxins on storage and release of neurotransmitters." In Harvey A (ed.). *Natural and Synthetic Neurotoxins.* Academic Press, San Diego, 1993, pp. 278–317.
3. Jankovic, J, Brin, MF. "Therapeutic uses of botulinum toxin." *N Engl J Med.* 1991 Apr 25;324(17):1186–94.
4. Halar, EM, Hammond, MC, Dirks, S. "Physical activity; its influence on nerve conduction velocity." *Arch Phys Med Rehabil.* 1985;66:605–9.
5. This file is licensed under the Creative Commons Attribution ShareAlike 2.5, Attribution ShareAlike 2.0 and Attribution ShareAlike 1.0 License.
6. Mcarthy, M, Jr, Chang, CH. Pickard, AS et al. "Visual analogue scales for assessing surgical pain." *J Am College Surg.* 2005;201(2):245–52.
7. Sellin, LC, Kauffman, JA, Dasgupta, BR. "Comparison of the effects of botulinum neurotoxin types A and E at the rat neuromuscular junction." *Med Biol.* 1983 Apr; 61(2):120–5.
8. Sellin, LC, Thesleff, S, Dasgupta, BR. "Different effects of types A and B botulinum toxin on transmitter release at the rat neuromuscular junction." *Acta Physiol Scand.* 1983;119(2): 127–33.

Chapter 6
Piriformis Syndrome: Electrophysiology *vs.* Anatomical Assumption

Abstract The FAIR-test for piriformis syndrome is the functional electrodiagnostic test which we have done the longest, and for which we have the best evidence. We have encountered stiff resistance and received many valuable suggestions during the 23 years we have used this test, many of which have helped shape the "flagship" test which this chapter describes. Recent advances in imaging techniques and cumulative surgical results have provided significant confirmation of the syndrome's pathogenetic mechanism as well as its high incidence in our sedentary, health-clubby civilization.

Keywords H loop · Gemellus major and minor · Obturator internus · Quadratus femoris · Sciatic nerve · Sural sensory · Denervation · Interference pattern · Neuropathy Herniated nucleus pulposus (HNP) · H-reflex delay

Can Piriformis Syndrome Be Operationally Defined?

Piriformis syndrome is another erstwhile diagnosis of exclusion that recently has been lifted from that status by a functional electrodiagnostic maneuver, and later verified by other means. Before Mixter and Barr [1] described spinal pathology as a basis for sciatica, that symptom was often ascribed to difficulties near the ischial bone, accounting for its earlier Italian name *ischiatica*. In earlier times Pott's disease, sacroiliac joint arthritis, and tubercular fistulae burrowing along the iliapsoas muscles were often held responsible for sciatica.

While Columbus was busy discovering the New World, the hospitals of Savanarola's fifteenth century Florence were ministering to many individuals suffering from sciatica, with therapy directed to ischial sites. Since then the pendulum has swung to the other extreme. The current combination of imaging studies, anesthetized and relatively infection-free surgery, and the medical growth-industry of lower back surgery have created a narrowly focused medical community that has trouble believing that sciatic pain could possibly result from anywhere except the lower spine! But sometimes a cigar is just a cigar, and it stands to reason that sometimes pain in the leg and buttock can originate in the buttock and leg.

L.M. Fishman, A.N. Wilkins, *Functional Electromyography*,
DOI 10.1007/978-1-60761-020-5_6,

There is, actually, good evidence for piriformis syndrome that has come to light in the past 20 years. However, it is difficult to estimate the incidence of a condition for which there are a number of different diagnostic criteria. In 1937, Friberg [2], a surgeon, gave the following three indications for piriformis-caused sciatica: [1] tenderness at the sciatic notch [2], positive Lasegue's sign, and [3] improvement with non-surgical treatment. Ten years later Robinson [3] delineated five salient characteristics [1]: history of local trauma [2]; pain localized to the sacroiliac joint, greater sciatic notch, and piriformis muscle, which extends along the course of the sciatic nerve and presents difficulty in walking [3]; acute pain brought on by stooping or lifting and relieved somewhat by traction [4]; palpable spindle or sausage-shaped mass at the anatomic location of the piriformis muscle; and [5] positive Lasegue's sign. Robinson also found gluteal atrophy more likely in piriformis syndrome.

But sacroiliac joint derangement and gluteal injections fit Freibergs's criteria, and Robinson's exacting list selects out all but a fraction of the piriformis syndrome cases identified clinically, even as a diagnosis of exclusion. Furthermore, no rationale was given by either investigator for these boundary rules. Finally, most clinical diagnoses were made through digital anal or vaginal examinations of patients who had already been "filtered" through a series of negative diagnostic tests. The shrouded figure of a diagnosis of exclusion hovered about piriformis syndrome, clouding over the possibility that a patient could have *both* a herniated disc, for example, and piriformis syndrome. Paradoxically, and illogically, no one doubted that a patient might have scarlet fever and piriformis syndrome, or fleas and lice.

In the last 50 years, a number of investigators have looked for and believed they found piriformis syndrome, almost always defined as entrapment of the sciatic nerve by that muscle [4–8]. Roger Hallin [9], investigating 910 successive cases entering the Mayo Clinic with sciatica, estimated piriformis syndrome be the cause of sciatica in 6% of the cases. He tested for it with rectal examinations. The registry in Olmstead County, Minnesota, [10] where the Mayo clinic is located, recorded 32,655 cases of lower back pain in the years 1976–2001. The diagnosis of piriformis syndrome was made 220 times over that period, giving a diagnostic rate of 0.7%. In 1976–1979, the diagnosis was made in 11 of 4,416 cases, a rate of 0.25%, whereas in 2000–2001 it was made in 54 of 4,349 cases (1.24%), showing nearly a fivefold rise over this quarter century, but still fivefold short of what was seen in an unbiased sample by experts at the Mayo Clinic. All these clinicians used rectal and vaginal examinations. Walter Reed Hospital [10] reported 155 cases of piriformis syndrome out of 9,161 diagnoses for low back pain (1.58%) during the year 2002.

In New York, we have seen more than 15,000 patients over the past 20 years who were suspected of having piriformis syndrome. Approximately half of them actually did. We more closely studied the past history of a select group of 918 patients who had piriformis syndrome. We could document 1,190 related MRIs, 1,380 related X-ray studies, 860 other imaging studies such as bone scans and ultrasonic examinations, and over 400 surgeries (spinal, hip, and gynecological, in that order), and very numerous other procedures such as epidural injections, prolotherapies, and nerve blocks. The average piriformis-positive patient saw 6.55 clinicians for sciatica over a period of 6.2 years before entering this study. MRIs of the lumbar spine were often done two, even three times, and multiple lower back surgeries were not rare. This suggests that many of the previous clinicians considered piriformis syndrome a diagnosis of exclusion or did not consider it at all.

In spite of its economic advantage, few doctors would consider rectal examination among their favorite tests. In any event, pain on this examination is far from pathognomonic for piriformis syndrome. A non-specific test justifies using an elaborate rule-out protocol before considering it definitive for any diagnosis. Yet data from the Mayo Clinic, Walter Reed Hospital, and our own (hardly unbiased) data, as well as the very logic of the idea of a "diagnosis of exclusion" all suggest that, in spite of this test and its built-in false positives, piriformis syndrome might be significantly underdiagnosed.

Recent developments in MRI technology and software have provided a type of imaging that tends to confirm this. By digitally subtracting the fat-suppression image from full MRI images of the pelvis, the fat-covered structures such as nerves are highlighted. While not as clear or quite as unequivocal as old-fashioned X rays are for bony pathology, the neural scans, as they have come to be known, reveal many features such as compression, inflammation, and actual nerve narrowing and flattening in precision and detail that were previously available only in surgery.

Dr. Filler et al. at Cedars-Sinai Hospital studied 239 patients, approximately half of whom had sciatica unrelieved by lumbar spinal surgery, and the other half of whom had too little MRI or standard EMG evidence for the surgery to be performed at all [11]. What they had in common was sciatica. Performing up to 30 of the neural scans on each of these patients, they reported strong evidence that more than two-thirds of them had piriformis muscle entrapment (see Fig. 6.1). In an article titled "Sciatica of nondisc origin and piriformis syndrome: diagnosis by magnetic resonance neurography and interventional magnetic of resonance imaging with outcome study of resulting treatment" [11], they also reported the percentages of other extra-spinal causes of sciatica:

Final diagnoses after evaluation and treatment in 239 patients with non-disc sciatica [11]

Diagnosis	Percent of patients
Piriformis syndrome	67.8
Distal foraminal entrapment	6.0
Ischial tunnel syndrome	4.7
no diagnosis	4.2
Discogenic pain with referred/referred leg pain	3.4
Pudendal nerve/sacrospinous ligament	3.0
Distal sciatic entrapment	2.1
Sciatic tumor	1.7
Lumbosacral plexus entrapment	1.3
Unappreciated lateral disc herniation	1.3

(continued)

Diagnosis	Percent of patients
Nerve root injury due to spinal operation	1.3
Inadequate spinal root decompression	0.8
Lumbar stenosis presenting as sciatica	0.8
Sacroiliac joint inflammation	0.8
Sacral fracture	0.4
Tumor in lumbosacral plexus	0.4

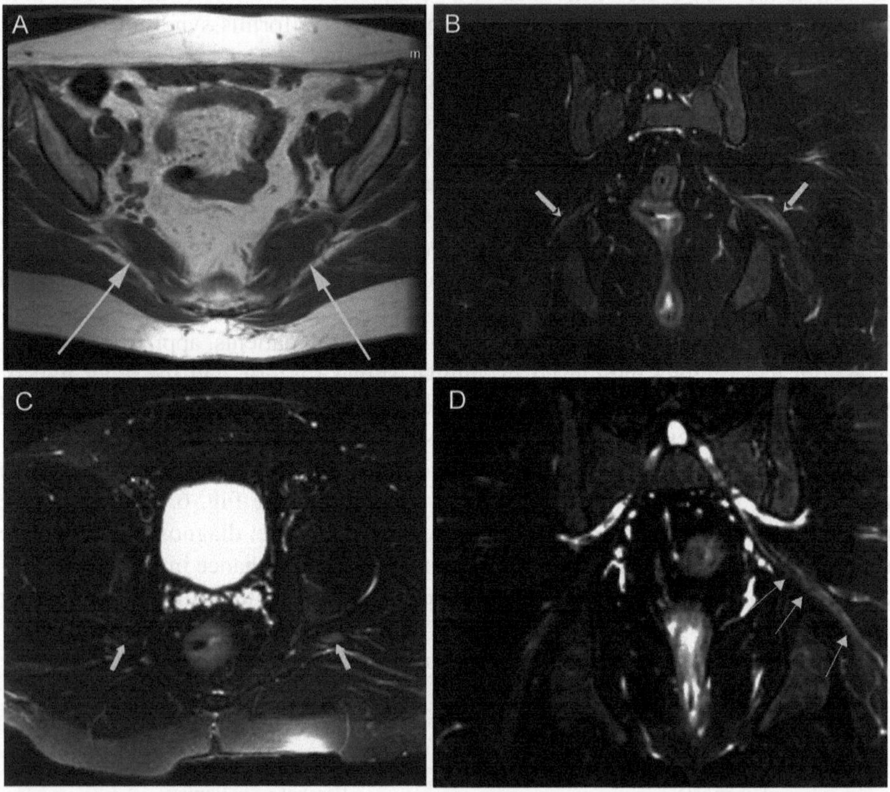

Fig. 6.1 Magnetic resonance neurography findings in piriformis syndrome. **a** Axial T1-weighted image of piriformis muscle size asymmetry (*arrows* indicate piriformis muscles). The left piriformis muscle is enlarged. **b**, **c** Coronal and axial images of the pelvis. *Arrows* indicate sciatic nerves. The left sciatic nerve exhibited hyperintensity. **d** Curved reformatted neurography image demonstrating left sciatic nerve hyperintensity and loss of fascicular detail at the sciatic notch (*arrows*). With the permission of Dr. Aaron Filler et al., p. 106 [11]

In that study, more than two-thirds of the patients, who had sciatica but no proven lumbar condition, had piriformis syndrome. Some had no evidence on MRI suggesting lumbar pathology; 49% had lumbar disc pathology sufficient to trigger spinal surgery that had no beneficial effect, since the cause of the sciatica, the pain generator, was not in the lumbar spine.

Questions of the actual incidence and prevalence of piriformis syndrome are only answerable in estimates. In view of the diversity of criteria used to identify it, any estimate must be viewed with caution.

Dr. Filler writes: "The true incidence of piriformis syndrome is not clear at this time. Lacking agreement even on the existence of the diagnosis and on how to establish the diagnosis if it does exist, epidemiological work has been scarce. The typical absence of a positive SLR sign, the presence of multidermatomal pain not extending to the toes, and the negative lumbar MR imaging may account for the low rate of referral of these patients to neurosurgeons and orthopedic spine specialists. The low rate of referral and frequent failure to recognize the diagnosis, however, should not be mistaken for evidence of a low incidence in the population.

"However, there is a reasonable inference to be made from the fact that of 1.5 million patients with sciatica severe enough to require MR imaging, only 200,000 proved to have a treatable herniated disc. One interpretation of the results obtained in our study population is that piriformis syndrome may be as common as herniated discs in the cause of sciatica.

"Because an accurate diagnosis is not established in more than 1 million patients with severe sciatica [80% of the total population receiving lumbosacral MRIs] each year when using the reference standard diagnostic paradigm, our new technologies and the expanded diagnostic criteria merit careful consideration by those primary and specialist physicians charged with the evaluation and management of these patients" [11].

Piriformis syndrome may be defined as sciatica-like symptoms caused by entrapment of fibers of the sciatic nerve by the piriformis muscle. But then again, what exactly is sciatica? The faddish association with lumbar spinal pathology has actually brought a number of American medical dictionaries to define sciatica as pain that is due to a specific spinal cause. For example, "Pain in the lower back and hip radiating down the back of the thigh into the leg, initially attributed to sciatic nerve dysfunction (hence the term), but now known to usually be due to herniated lumbar disk compromising a nerve root, most commonly the L5 or S1 root." (Stedman's Medical Dictionary, 27th Edition), but that is misleading.

Sciatica is a symptom, not an illness, though it is a symptom-with-a-set-of-causes. The symptoms should be in the course of the sciatic nerve, and, if they actually are from nerve root or cauda equina rootlet pathology, should conform to the dermatomes, myotomes, sclerotomes, and osteotomes of the lumbar spine. If the cause is distal to the joining of the roots in the lumbosacral plexus, then the pattern of symptoms will relate to the destinations of the more peripheral fiber-grouping of the sciatic nerve at the level of the injury. Intermittent claudication, multiple sclerosis, and even CVA may mimic sciatica, but they are not; the first of these conditions even being nicknamed "pseudosciatica."

In the case of piriformis syndrome, the symptoms are often distributed along the course of the peroneal and/or posterior tibial branches of the sciatic nerve, sometimes affecting one branch in all its peripheral ramiculations, but not necessarily the other. The entrapment itself is usually brought about by extensive and prolonged sitting, and it is seen most in secretaries and psychiatrists, bankers and bus drivers, serious students and others who spend sedentary days, but there are other common causes. Runners, especially runners in training for marathons, health-club devotees, blunt or not-so-blunt trauma, occurring in automobile accidents and backward falls, misplaced hypodermic injections or deep lacerations, extreme obesity or asthenia, and, rarely, anatomical causes such as muscle–nerve interpenetration, anomalous course of the inferior gluteal artery or vein, or spondylolisthesis, this latter not infrequently causing spasm of extensor muscles and the piriformis.

Gardenpathogenesis

One seductive but spurious explanation for piriformis syndrome involves the common anatomical variants. Approximately 15% of the time, one or both branches of the sciatic nerve pass through or even over the piriformis muscle (Table 6.1 and Fig. 6.2).

It is not uncommon for the posterior and anterior divisions of the lumbosacral plexus to remain ununited, and pass by the piriformis muscle and through the ischial tunnel separately. This might appear to be a likely explanation for entrapment there. However, in the anatomy lab at Albert Einstein College of Medicine, we looked at 76 cadavers, finding that these anatomical anomalies were invariably bilateral, yet piriformis syndrome is unilateral 90% of the time. Friberg and Sunderland, in anatomical studies, found the peroneal branch of the sciatic nerve anomalous in 75% of these cases, yet the posterior division (that becomes the posterior tibial nerve) is more frequently and more seriously involved in piriformis syndrome [12–14]. Furthermore, following 80 confirmed cases through surgery, we found the incidence of these anomalies to be just about 15%: no greater than what was seen in the general (cadaveric) population. Still further, though this gets a little ahead of our story, the syndrome may be cured more than 80% of the time without doing anything to the structural anatomy. The surgery, usually a neurolysis, has had close to the same 80% success rate on the 120 of our conservative treatment failures that have had recourse to it in the past 20 years.

Table 6.1 In Europe and the United States, the following studies confirm that the usual anatomical variants, penetration of the muscle by one or both divisions of the sciatic nerve's components occurs in 15% to 20% of cases, usually when the divisions do not unite distal to the lumbosacral plexus, which is estimated to occur 25–33% of the time

Author (year)	Specimens	% Variation
Yeoman (1928)	100	20
Pecina (1979)	130	21.5
Beaton (1983)	120	10.0
Gotlin (1990)	42	16.7
Fishman (2000)	76	17.8

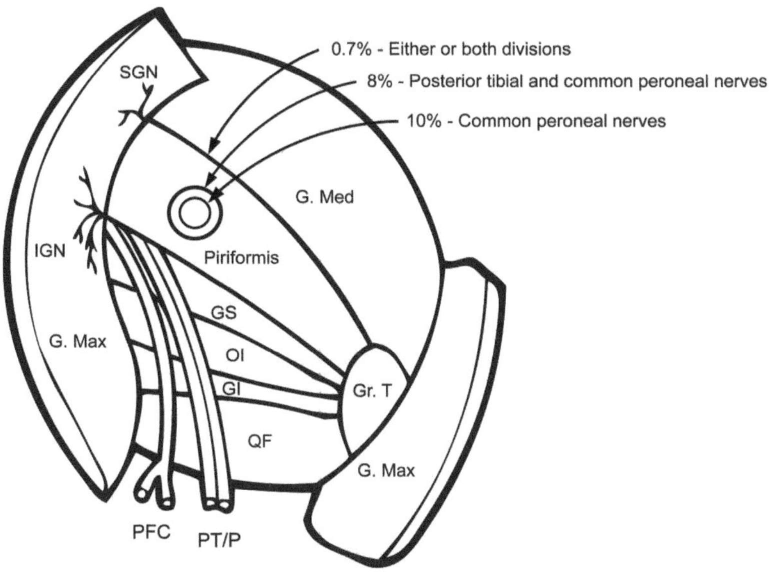

Fig. 6.2 Muscles: G. max. = gluteus maximus; G. med. = gluteus medius; GS = gemellus superior; OI = obturator internis; GI = gemellus inferior; QF = quadratus femoris. Nerves: SGN = superior gluteal nerve; IGN = inferior gluteal nerve; PFC = posterior femoral cutaneous; PT/P = posterior tibial and peroneal. The superior and inferior gluteal arteries travel with the nerves of the same name; the inferior gluteal artery occasionally entraps one or both branches of the sciatic nerve at the greater sciatic foramen

Some Cadaveric Studies of Anomalous Sciatic-Piriformis Intersection

The Anatomy Close-Up

One of the strongest arguments against Intelligent Design is the ischiofemoral ligament, a sharp-edged collagenous structure that runs just below the piriformis muscle and deep into it. The sciatic nerve descends between them, and may be compressed by the muscle and lacerated by the ligament. Spasm or unusually strong or prolonged pressure on the muscle will force the nerve against the sharp, obdurate edge of the ligament, causing entrapment and possibly damage to the epineurium, and in some instances to the perineurium, endoneurium, and the nerve fibers themselves (Fig. 6.3).

Although pressure is usually intermittent, and related to position, the damage can be structural and enduring. Approximately 10% of the cases we have encountered display some peripheral denervation, usually in the gastrocnemius or anterior tibialis. Generally the patients' pain subsists at a lower level until sitting or other provocative conditions amplify it, often considerably. One theory of causation suggests that certain people's genomic profile renders them more vulnerable

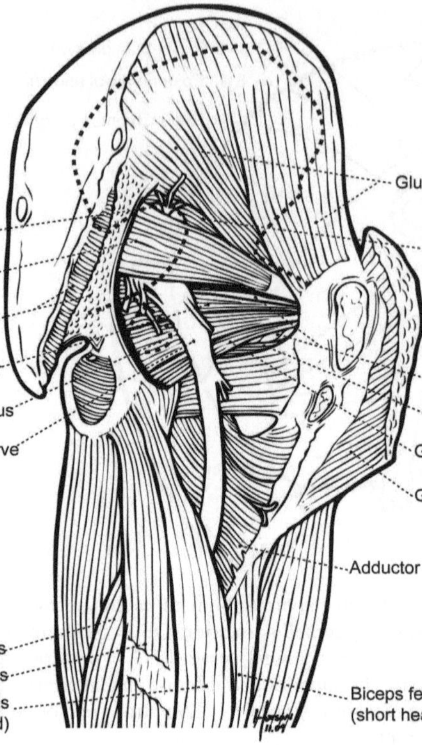

Fig. 6.3 The sciatic nerve exits the pelvis just below the piriformis muscle, and just superficial to the ischiofemoral ligament, then passing superficial to the gemelli, obturator internus and quadratus femoris, and finally through the ischial tunnel to the proximal thigh

to the stresses and strains of contemporary sedentary and health-club life. This might be the forme fruste of a myelin abnormality of the sort that causes Charcot Marie-Tooth, only significantly less severe: this vulnerability may be so slight that without particular environmental stimulus, the matter would remain subclinical. Asymmetrical or (less frequently) symmetrical, intensification of these stresses is then all it takes to bring about the syndrome [15].

Symptoms

The strongest symptoms of piriformis syndrome are buttock tenderness and pain, numbness, paraesthesias and/or weakness in the distribution of the sciatic nerve and its branches. The pattern of numbness and the other symptoms is usually according to the anatomy of the posterior tibial and peroneal nerves, rather than following a dermatomal pattern. Some students of the syndrome [11] note numbness of the toes rather than the feet as less characteristic of piriformis syndrome than sciatica's other causes. An importantly common but not ubiquitous feature is that pain is worsened by pressure on the buttock and by sitting or lying supine.

Tenderness should be greatest at the intersection of the sciatic nerve and the piriformis muscle, where the compression occurs. The only problem with this straightforward association is that the buttock itself has few landmarks; it is not always so easy to find that intersection, especially in obese patients. Guided by two recognizable points, the proximal tip of the greater trochanter and the greater sciatic notch, one can palpate for any tender spots on, above, or below a horizontal triangle with apex at the greater trochanter that widens to 4–6 cm at the sciatic foramen. The actual intersection of muscle and nerve is usually in the middle third of that band. In slender people, light palpation finds a medially and slightly rostrally inclined bevel in the buttock that widens as one traces it medially from the greater trochanter to the sciatic notch and is the piriformis muscle.

Signs

When it comes to signs, we have found that the straight leg raise (SLR) is generally positive, but not at all specific. We generally take it as positive when there is a 15° side-to-side discrepancy, or absolute value below 60° in bilateral cases. It may raise suspicion of piriformis syndrome if the pain SLR generates is in the buttock rather than the lower back, and if there is no contralateral pain of any kind. But the SLR is neither a necessary nor a sufficient condition; as an indicator of piriformis syndrome, it is not really very persuasive. We have definitely seen cases with negative straight leg raise.

Weakened abduction of the flexed thigh, first described in the *Western Journal of Medicine* by Pace [8], is certainly the most commonly positive sign in piriformis syndrome and a strong indicator of its presence. Since the piriformis muscle is a tertiary abductor of the flexed thigh, the weakness may be due to reflex inhibition of abduction mediated at the spinal level rather than any actual weakness of the piriformis muscle. In fact, its strength in compressing the sciatic nerve appears to be the pathogenetic mechanism.

Buttock pain with passive adduction of the flexed thigh, first described by the Norwegian neurosurgeon Solheim [16], is also sometimes observed in piriformis syndrome. The same maneuver may often bring pain in the hip and inguinal region, but those are quite different, and are usually due to trochanteric bursitis and hip pathology, respectively.

Sometimes these maneuvers or pressure in the region of intersection of the piriformis muscle and the sciatic nerve actually produce sciatic-like symptoms. This, of course, is highly suggestive of piriformis entrapment of the sciatic nerve. It is also a clinical rendition of the functional electrodiagnostic test that forms the heart of this chapter.

Electrophysiological Suggestion of Piriformis Syndrome

The electromyographer may begin to consider alternative causes when a patient with sciatica gives no evidence of paraspinal denervation. Naturally, there are radiculopathies with only anterior primary division injury, but they are in a decided minority of cases with radiculopathic involvement. Doubt of a classical radiculopathy may creep in when paraspinal examination fails to reveal any abnormalities.

1. Of course in *simple* cases of piriformis syndrome, there is never any paraspinal denervation, but its absence, though part of the picture, is hardly definitive. Although radiculopathy must be excluded to firmly identify piriformis syndrome as *the* cause of sciatica in any given case, we have actually found a number of individuals in whom piriformis syndrome coexists with other conditions such as radiculopathy, and for example, sacroiliac joint derangement. As we have been insisting, piriformis syndrome is not a diagnosis of exclusion, but has criteria for its own identification.
2. *Peroneal or posterior tibial pattern of peripheral denervation*, where injury to fibers of one division of the lumbosacral plexus is the simplest explanation. For example, one might suspect piriformis syndrome with positive sharp waves in the peroneus longus, brevis, tertius, and the anterior tibialis, but in neither gastrocnemius nor posterior tibialis nor plantar intrinsics.
3. *Involvement of lower extremities but not the hamstrings, nor the glutei nor the tensa fascie latae,* since the superior and inferior gluteal nerves do not travel with the sciatic nerve, and the nervous supply to the hamstrings usually breaks free of the sciatic nerve proximal to the piriformis muscle. Rare exceptions to these muscles' uninvolvement may be seen with blunt trauma, misplaced gluteal injections, and hemorrhages near the lumbosacral plexus, e.g., related to placement of a Greenfield filter.
4. *Reduction of sural sensory nerve action potential on the affected side*, suggesting an injury distal to the ganglia.

Mix of Clinical and Electrophysiological Findings

Unsurprisingly, sometimes a combination of clinical and electrophysiological findings will suggest piriformis syndrome, such as denervation in the anterior tibialis without sensory disturbances in the medial calf or profound weakness in abduction of the flexed thigh without denervation of lumbar paraspinals or the primary abductors themselves.

Functional Confirmation: Electrophysiological Evidence of Piriformis Syndrome

But to really diagnose piriformis syndrome, we need more than an index of suspicion. We need a test in which the independent variable is tightness of the piriformis muscle on the sciatic nerve, and the dependent variable is change in sciatic nerve function. Clinically, this is pain, numbness, or paraesthesias directly appearing in the flexed, adducted internally rotated (FAIR) position. Electrophysiologically it is significant impairment in sciatic nerve conduction during that provocative maneuver.

If the piriformis muscle exerts significant compressive force on the sciatic nerve, then placing patients with the syndrome in the FAIR position should tighten the muscle sufficiently to compress the sciatic nerve's fibers and transiently slow nerve conduction past that point. If we use the H reflex, then the difference between the anatomical and FAIR-position's total conduction time should be enhanced by the fact that the afferent and the efferent limbs of the reflex cross and re-cross the muscle, thereby amplifying any discrepancy that the tightening generates by a factor of 2 [14].

We published a small article about 37 patients confirming the above fact in the *Archives of Physical Medicine and Rehabilitation* in 1992 [12] that received attention in the lay press. The exposure drew patients to our offices from all parts of the globe. Approximately 75% lived in New York, Connecticut, New Jersey, or Pennsylvania. Another 20% came from other American urban centers, and 5% came from North and South America, Europe, Asia, Africa, and Australia.

Serial patients presenting with low back pain or sciatica were classified as having piriformis syndrome if they met at least two of the following three clinical criteria [1]: pain at the intersection of the piriformis muscle and the sciatic nerve (the site of the pathology) in the FAIR position (see Fig. 6.2)) [2]; tenderness at the intersection of the piriformis muscle and the sciatic nerve (mechanical pressure replicating the pathogenetic mechanism), and/or [3] positive supine Lasegue's sign, taken as a 15° reduction in painless straight leg raise on the affected *vs.* the unaffected side or less than 60° in bilateral cases. At that point we believed that SLR would tend to intensify compression by sandwiching the nerve between the ischiofemoral ligament and the piriformis muscle.

We recorded detailed histories and did detailed physical examinations and follow-ups on 918 patients complaining of lower back pain and/or sciatica in whom 1,014 limbs were involved (96 cases were bilateral).

Each patient was placed in the anatomical position, and unilateral or bilateral posterior tibial and peroneal H reflexes were sought. We conducted posterior tibial H-reflex testing according to the guidelines described by Hugon [17] and Braddom and Johnson [18]. Peroneal H reflexes were elicited by placing a bar electrode 6 cm distal to the fibular head and stimulating at the lateral popliteal fossa. Gain was set at 500 mV, and filters were set at 100–10,000 Hz, with sweep at 5 ms/division. Limb temperature, pre-examination exercise, and timing of successive H-reflex stimuli were taken into account throughout the work, according to the guidelines of Bell and Lehman [19] and Halar et al. [20].

Technique

Patients were then placed in the FAIR position (Fig. 6.4), being careful to adduct the leg. If one pushes straight down in adducting the upper leg of a patient in lateral

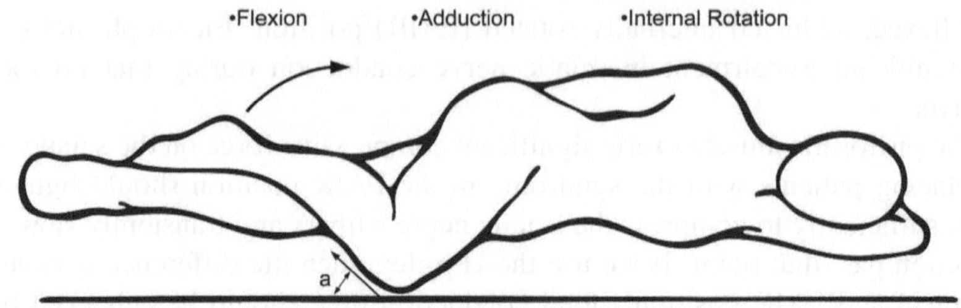

Fig. 6.4 We press the superior knee and hip backward as well as downward to maximize adduction while increasing the angle of internal rotation (a)

decubitus, he or she might simply tilt the pelvis forward, actually placing the leg in abduction by the time the knee comes down to the examination table. Better to follow this protocol: one positions the patient in lateral decubitus facing the examiner; then the examiner pushes the lateral knee of the upper (examined) leg toward the contralateral groin, on a downward diagonal, actually controlling pelvic motion through this angling of the upper hip, and preventing any forward movement of the patient's pelvis toward the examiner.

Many of the people being tested do, naturally, have tight and tender piriformis muscles, which prompts them to resist this effort, and require a firm but considerate approach to this admittedly provocative maneuver. Almost all patients can sustain sufficient flexion, adduction, and internal rotation to significantly prolong the H reflex, or to convince the examiner that significant pressure of the piriformis muscle on the sciatic nerve or its branches is not inducible through this means.

Technical Metrics

H reflexes were elicited again, observing the same guidelines. FAIR-position H reflexes were elicited within 5 s of patients' arriving at the correct position, and the greatest twice-replicable latencies were recorded. A rest interval of 5 or more seconds separated one FAIR-test positioning and testing from the next, minimizing the effect of repetitive stimulation on H-reflex latency [21, 22]. H reflexes and M waves of similar configuration were recorded in anatomic and FAIR positions for both nerves.

The legs of 44 asymptomatic individuals were tested on a different occasion following the same procedure [12]. An additional 44 legs of asymptomatic volunteers were tested, bringing the total to 88. The standard deviation (SD) of these normal legs' H-reflex latencies' delay in the FAIR position was used to gauge abnormality in suspected cases of piriformis syndrome. For comparison, contralateral legs of 229 FAIR-test positive (FTP) patients were tested according to the same protocol.

Measurement of Delay: The H Loop

To account for any subcutaneous nerve movements that might occur when patients changed from the anatomic to the FAIR position, we calculated the entire reflex arc's latency by taking the sum of the distal motor latency or M wave from the point of stimulation in the popliteal fossa to the soleus or peroneus longus muscle, plus the H-reflex latency, forming what might be called an H loop analogous to the F loop calculations usually made for F waves in the upper extremities. Movement of the point along the nerve at which stimulation takes place has no effect on the latency of the H loop except that the sensory limb of the H reflex is made shorter (or longer) by the same distance that the path of the distal motor latency is lengthened (or shortened). This will only change the latency if the motor and sensory nerve conduction velocities are disparate.

Discrepancy Between Motor and Sensory Nerve Conduction Velocity

One can estimate the range of built-in difference in the FAIR test assuming a 5-cm movement of the sciatic nerve and a 10 meters/second (m/s) discrepancy between motor and sensory nerve conduction velocities (NCV) with the following formula:

$$D/R = T$$

$$0.05\,\text{m}/50\,\text{m/s} = 0.001\,\text{s}$$

$$0.5\,\text{m}/40\,\text{m/s} = 0.00125\,\text{s}$$

The difference in H loop will be 0.00025 s for every 10 m/s discrepancy between motor and sensory NCV, given a 5-cm movement of the sciatic nerve. If a 10 m/s discrepancy between motor (50 m/s) and sensory (40 m/s) NCV were present, then a 5-cm movement of the sciatic nerve's stimulation point would entail a 0.25 ms change in the sum of M + H latencies. This is less than one half of one SD in our study (see Figs. 6.5, 6.6, and 6.7).

To put this in perspective, a 20 m/s difference between motor and sensory NCV, and a 5-cm movement of the nerve beneath the skin would contribute less than one standard deviation change in the H loop. Because motor and sensory NCV are nearly equal in normal circumstances, the point of stimulation is generally immaterial to H loop values (see Fig. 6.5).

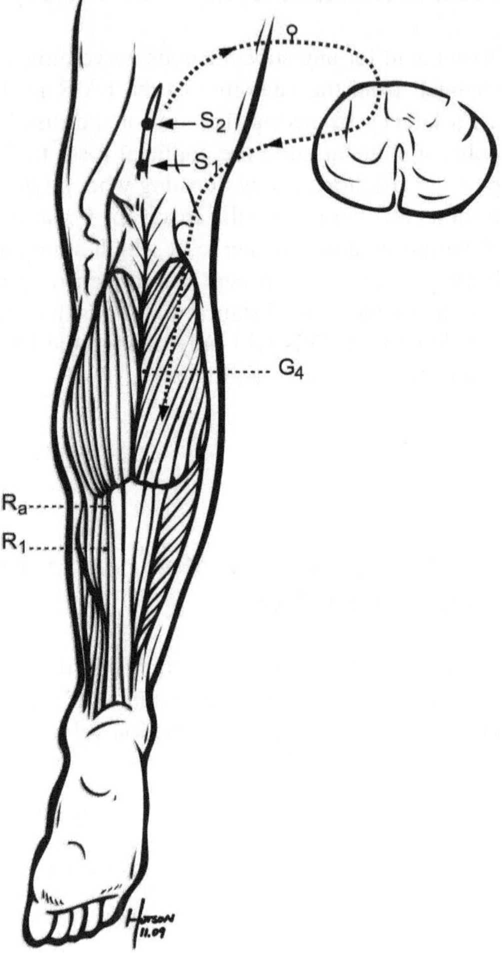

Fig. 6.5 If the point of H reflex stimulation is moved from S1 to S2, then the afferent limb of the reflex will be shortened by S2–S1. However, the distance that the M wave travels will be lengthened by the same amount. Only if the *discrepancy* in nerve conduction velocity between sensory (afferent limb of H reflex) and motor (motor limb of H reflex + M-wave latency) neurons were above 60 m/s, or the sciatic nerve moved 30 cm would this generate a significant prolongation in the H-reflex latencies of the magnitude observed in FAIR *vs.* anatomical positions

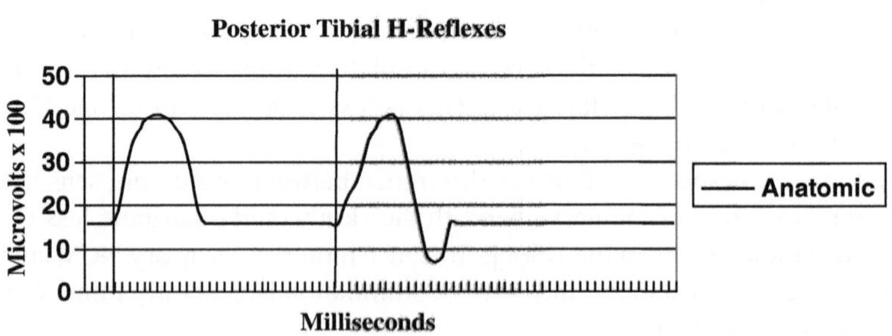

Fig. 6.6 The H loop (M wave plus H reflex) gives the timing from the point of stimulation down to the soleus and of stimulation through the synapse at the anterior horn and back down to the soleus

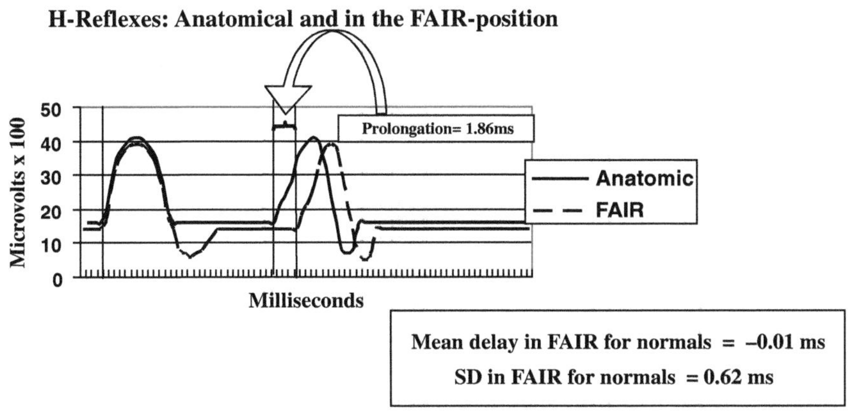

Fig. 6.7 The sciatic nerve might move when the piriformis muscle is stretched across it. Measuring the H loop accounts for that movement; a significant prolongation of the H loop (3 SD = 1.86 ms) indicates piriformis entrapment

Results

Although configuration of the H-reflex tracing was geometrically similar for the anatomic position and the FAIR position in each nerve tested, H-reflex amplitude often varied and tended toward reduction in piriformis syndrome patients in the FAIR position. When compression turned out to be significant, it was often necessary to raise stimulus intensity, possibly due to some fibers' reduced conduction velocity and the effect of this on temporal summation. Not rarely, though, a Jendrassic-like effect required lowering the stimulus intensity to obtain a maximal H reflex when the buttock muscles were stretched, and the reflex's amplitude was sometimes enhanced.

Maximum FAIR-test values for H reflexes obtained in 88 normal persons (asymptomatic controls) showed mean delay of −0.01 ms beyond values obtained in the anatomic position, with SD equal to 0.62 ms (see Table 6.2).

Patients meeting two of the three clinical criteria for piriformis syndrome had mean overall FAIR-test H-reflex prolongation of 3.39 and 3.11 ms for the posterior tibial and peroneal nerves, respectively. These values were 5.45 and 5.02 SD beyond the mean for the FAIR tests of asymptomatic individuals. Legs of patients with back pain and/or sciatica but failing to meet two of three clinical criteria for piriformis syndrome had average FAIR-test prolongation of 0.83 ms, 1.34 SD beyond the normal mean ($P < 0.001$) (see Table 6.2) [14].

A delay ≥3 SD on the FAIR test (1.86 ms) was seen in posterior tibial and or peroneal nerves in 468 of 537 limbs of patients meeting two of three clinical criteria for piriformis syndrome and in 22 of 151 limbs of patients who did not meet two of three clinical criteria. This showed a sensitivity of 0.881 and a specificity of 0.832. A delay of 2 SD (1.24 ms) was seen in 518 of 537 patients meeting two of three

Table 6.2 Validity of the FAIR test[a]

Piriformis syndrome[b]	Yes	No	Total
Positive FAIR test	512	69	581
Negative FAIR test	26	129	155
Total	538	198	736

[a]H-reflex prolonged more than 3 SD beyond the mean (1.86 ms) by flexion, adduction and internal rotation (FAIR test).
[b]Met at least two of the three clinical criteria.
Sensitivity, 0.881; specificity, 0.832.

criteria and in 44 of 151 patients' legs who did not. At 2 SDs, the FAIR test had a sensitivity of 0.968 and specificity of 0.686 (Table 6.2) [14].

In an obvious sense, the contralaterals are well-matched controls. Notably, however, the contralateral posterior tibial and peroneal FAIR tests of FTP patients (in unilateral cases) showed mean delay of 0.93 and 0.51 ms, respectively. This finding was significant in comparison with normal limbs ($P < 0.001$). This may suggest a systemic vulnerability to compression, e.g., changes in myelin composition, or common exposure to compression of both sciatic nerves, e.g., in sitting, running, and bilateral trauma.

The ipsilateral and contralateral posterior tibial branches were more frequently and more severely affected than the peroneal branches according to the FAIR test (Fig. 6.8).

At this point we have gone about as far as we can to show the efficacy of functional EMG in making a diagnosis that can be corroborated or contested by neural scanning MRI. In practice, over the past 3 years, we have sent 25 patients whom we believed to have piriformis syndrome down to the neural scanner in Norristown, Pennsylvania. These patients had positive FAIR tests but were not responding to

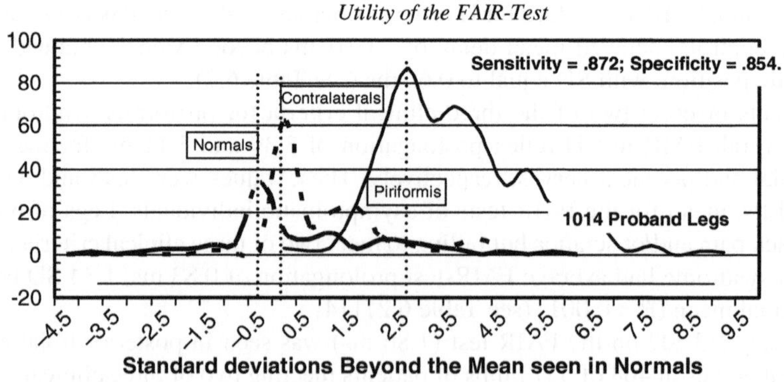

Fig. 6.8 Frequency distribution of FAIR-test values of patients with clinical piriformis syndrome, individual nerves of legs contralateral to clinical piriformis syndrome legs, and normals. Distance on the vertical axis is a measure of frequency. The horizontal axis extends from –4.5 to +11.5 ms in terms of standard deviations. 1 SD = 0.62 ms

treatment. It was natural to doubt our diagnosis, and the neural scanner seemed a good way to resolve or validate that doubt. In response, 24 of 25 had evidence of piriformis syndrome; the 25th patient had ischial tunnel compression, which, in the study of "non-disc sciatica" was seen in 4.7% of cases [11].

References

1. Mixter, WJ, Barr, JS. "Rupture of the intervertebral disc with involvement of the spinal canal." *New Engl J Med.* 1934;211:210.
2. Friberg, AH, Vinke, TH. "Sciatica and the sacro-iliac joint." *JBJS.* 1934;16:126–36.
3. Robinson, DR. "Piriformis syndrome in relation to sciatic pain." *Am J Surg.* 1947;73: 355–8.
4. Mizuguchi, T. "Division of the piriformis muscle for the treatment of sciatica. Postlaminectomy syndrome and osteoarthritis of the spine." *Arch Surg.* 1976 Jun;111(6): 719–22.
5. Childers, MK, Wilson, DJ, Gnatz, SM, Conway, RR, Sherman, AL. "Botulinum toxin in piriformis muscle syndrome." *Am J Phys Med Rehabil.* 2002;81:751–9.
6. Foster, MR. "Piriformis syndrome." *Orthopedics.* 2002;25:821–5.
7. Broadhurst, NA, Simmons, DN, Bond, MJ. "Piriformis syndrome: Correlation of muscle morphology with symptoms and signs." *Arch Phys Med Rehabil.* 2004 Dec;85(12):2036–9.
8. Pace, JB, Nagle, D. "Piriformis syndrome." *West J Med.* 1976;124:435–9.
9. Hallin, RP. "Sciatic pain and the piriformis muscle." *Postgrad Med.* 1983;74(69):72.
10. Fishman, LM, Schaefer, MP. "The piriformis syndrome is underdiagnosed." *Muscle Nerve.* 2003 Nov;28:646–9.
11. Filler, AG, Haynes, J, Jordan, SE, Prager, J, Villablanca, P, Farahani, K, McBride, DQ, Tsuruda, JS, Morisoli, B, Batzdorf, U, Johnson, JP. "Sciatica of nondisc origin and piriformis syndrome:diagnosis by magnetic resonance neurography and interventional magnetic resonance imaging with outcome study of resulting treatment." *J Neurosurg Spine.* 2005;2: 99–115.
12. Fishman, LM, Zybert, PA. "Electrophysiologic evidence of piriformis syndrome." *Arch Phys Med Rehabil.* 1992 Apr;73(4):359–64.
13. Fishman, L, Ardman, C. *Relief is in the Stretch.* W.W. Norton. New York, 2005.
14. Fishman, LM, Dombi, GW, Michaelsen, C, Ringel, SV, Rosbruch, J, Rosner, B, Weber, C. "Piriformis Syndrome: Diagnosis, treatment and outcome – a ten year study." *Arch Phys Med Rehabil.* 2002;83(3):295–302.
15. Kamholz, J, Awatramani, R, Menichella, D, Jiang, H, Xu, W, Shy, M. "Regulation of myelin-specific gene expression. Relevance to CMTI." Shy ME, Kamholz J, Lovelace RE (eds.). *Charcot-Marie-Tooth Disorders.* Vol. 883. Annals of the New York Academy of Sciences, New York, 1984, pp. 91–108.
16. Solheim, LF, Siewers, P, Paus, B. "The piriformis muscle syndrome. Sciatic nerve entrapment treated with section of the piriformis muscle." *Acta Orthop Scand.* 1981 Feb;52(1):73–5.
17. Hugon, M. "Methodology of the Hoffmann Reflex in man." In *New Developments in Elecxtromyography and Chemical Neurophysiology.* Desmedt JE, (ed.) Karger, Basel, 1973, pp. 227–93.
18. Braddom, RI, Johnson, EW. "Standardization of H reflex and T-reflexes in normal subjects." *Arch Phys Med Rehabil.* 1974;55:161–6.
19. Bell, KR, Lehmann, JF. "Effects of cooling on H- and T-reflexes in normal subjects." *Arch Phys Med Rehabil.* 1987;68:490–3.
20. Haler, EM, Hammond, MC, Dirks, S. "Physical activity: its influence on nerve conduction velocity." *Arch Phys Med Rehabil.* 1985;66:605–9.
21. Toth, S. "Frequency resonance investigation of the H-reflex." *J Neurol Psych.* 1979;42:351–6.
22. Hagbarth, K-E. "Post-tetanic potentiation of myotatic reflexes in man." *J Neurol Psych.* 1962;25:1–10.

Chapter 7
Treating Piriformis Syndrome Identified by a Provoked Electromyographic Sign: Analysis of the Data

Abstract Having isolated a test with prima facie relevance to entrapment of the sciatic nerve by the piriformis muscle, we review the success of treatment focused on that pathogenetic mechanism. The FAIR test's sensitivity and specificity are calibrated. We then investigate whether the functional test is a better predictor of successful treatment than positive signs and symptoms. Some further support for the functional test's utility may be seen in the correlation between the amount of delay seen in the FAIR test and patients' clinical improvement on the VAS.

Keywords Overdiagnosis · Underdiagnosis · Characteristics of piriformis syndrome · Contralateral · Odds ratio · Utility · Surgery · Myoneural junction · EMG guidance

Treatment of Piriformis Syndrome Patients Identified by Functional EMG

In an article titled "The piriformis syndrome is overdiagnosed," John Stewart [1], a neurosurgeon at McGill University, proposed that "ideally, the following five criteria need to be fulfilled to define such a [piriformis] syndrome:"

1. Presence of symptoms and signs of sciatic nerve damage.
2. Presence of electrophysiological evidence of sciatic nerve damage.
3. Imaging of the lumbosacral nerve roots and of the paravertebral and pelvic areas must be normal to exclude radiculopathy, or lower lumbar and sacral plexus infiltration or damage.
4. Surgical exploration of the proximal sciatic nerve should confirm an absence of mass lesions. *Ideally, compression of the sciatic nerve by the piriformis muscle or associated fibrous bands should be identified. However, it can sometimes be difficult to recognize a compressed nerve* [visually].
5. Relief of symptoms and improvement in neurological abnormalities should follow surgical decompression

L.M. Fishman, A.N. Wilkins, *Functional Electromyography*,
DOI 10.1007/978-1-60761-020-5_7,

This is not a flawless set. Obvious vestiges of "diagnosis of exclusion" are evident in refs [3]. and [4].

- Paraspinal and pelvic muscle electromyography (EMG) must be normal to exclude a radiculopathy.
- Surgical exploration should confirm an absence of mass lesions.

If one is doing research on piriformis syndrome, then yes, it is important to exclude other conditions that might confound outcome studies. But in life, things are complex. One can have two things at the same time. Failure to exclude hepatitis does not change a diagnosis of gall stones. Oat-cell tumor does not exclude tuberculosis.

The rest of Stewart's set also errs on the side of conservatism:

- There is no real necessity for sciatic nerve *damage* as suggested in ref [1]. either. In carpal tunnel and pronator syndrome, *symptoms* such as paraesthesias and pain, and/or *signs* such as weakness and sensory deficit, that are confirmed by nerve conduction slowing and thereby traceable to nerve compression are sufficient. That is the case here too.
- Relief of symptoms with surgery (item 5), as Dr. Stewart actually concedes in his article, is not really essential to the diagnosis of any compression neuropathy. Neither is it essential to the diagnosis of cancer, fracture, or anything else, that symptoms are removed with surgery though such relief might help determine which of several conditions is causing the patient's symptoms.

The second part of ref [4]. is quite relevant to our subject (italics and brackets put in by the authors), since functional EMG, where conduction is tested in a provocative position, is exactly intended to turn up pathology that is not structural, where there are no anatomical signs nor visible changes. Dr. Stewart warns that this might be difficult in the second italicized sentence: *However, it can sometimes be difficult to recognize a compressed nerve.* "Indeed, it might be nearly impossible, since the pathology is in the dynamic changes that occur with movement, and any motionless, conventional study, structural or electromyographic, for that matter . . . almost any study,[1] that fails to quantify the neurophysiological, functional changes that take place with changes in position, is almost certain to overlook. This, of course, is what we are attempting to evaluate.

Equally obvious is the only one of Dr. Stewart's criteria that is left standing, number [2], "Presence of electrophysiological evidence of sciatic nerve damage," and the fact that conventional electromyographic studies pick up only the most severe and egregious examples of piriformis syndrome, where

[1] Histological changes may appear.

compression had gone on long enough or progressed far enough to produce denervation.

In the last chapter, we effectively identified a group of patients characterized by reversible electrophysiological changes in the sciatic nerve when the tension of the piriformis muscle was increased. This group of patients, all with sciatica, was contrasted with controls who had no sciatica and did not show changes in the sciatic nerve's conduction with the same positional provocation. The question now is whether an individual's inclusion in the group showing electrophysiological changes has any bearing on what is causing his or her sciatica.

To persuasively single out a group of patients having delay in an electrophysiological version of a provocative maneuver has little clinical value unless it gives some guidance toward effective treatment. The class of "Midwestern poets with a high instep," might be reasonably delineated, but what would be the point? If we are to illustrate that a functional nerve conduction test has clinical value, we must show correlation between that test's results and the efficacy of treatment directed toward the likely determinants of the test's outcome.

Outcome Statistics of the 1,014 Leg Study

We followed, recorded, and analyzed the longer term course of the 918 patients in the study we described in Chapter 6 [2]. Approximately 10% had the condition bilaterally.

Treatment

Each patient who had H-loop latency prolongation beyond 1.86 ms, three standard deviations beyond the mean prolongation seen in 88 normals, or had two of the three clinical criteria, or for whom there was a high index of suspicion for piriformis syndrome, was treated according to the following two-part protocol [2].

1. *Injection*: A solution containing 1.5 ml of 2% lidocaine and 0.5 ml containing 20 mg triamcinolone acetonide was injected at a point one-third the distance from the greater trochanter to the area of maximum tenderness in the piriformis muscle at a depth of approximately 2.5–5 cm (see Fig. 7.1). This point, just medial to the musculotendinous junction, approximates the motor point of the piriformis muscle. Electromyographic localization of the piriformis muscle, now a standard procedure for the authors, was something we had just begun to do. We did it only when the muscle's uncertain location or depth required it.

Consenting patients received injections at the initial diagnostic visit. Repeat injections were done infrequently on patients judged to have insufficient improvement and on the average were given 6 weeks after the first injection.

2. *Concentrated physical therapy*: Patients were treated according to a standard protocol.

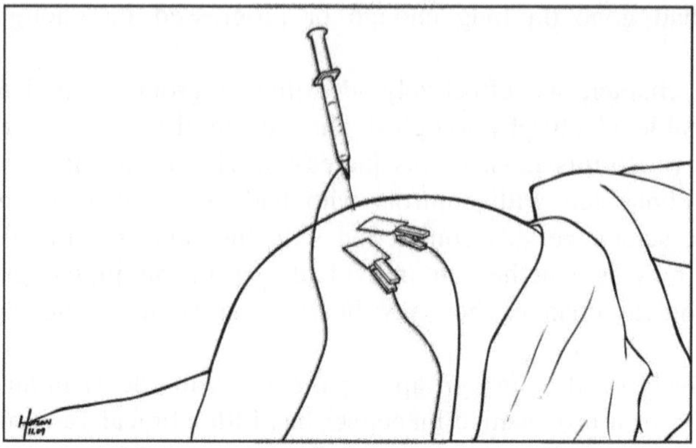

Fig. 7.1 The wedge-shaped piriformis muscle may be felt just beneath the gluteus maximus. When injecting lidocaine or marcaine and steroid, we selected a spot one-third the distance from the greater trochanter to the point of maximum tenderness on the theory that the tender point is most likely where the sciatic nerve crosses under the muscle. We have had no mishaps in more than 13,000 injections, and have had 11 cases of very temporary drop foot. Six of these occurred within the first 300 injections

Physical Therapy for Piriformis Syndrome*

1. Place patient in contralateral decubitus and *F*lexed *A*dducted *I*nternally *R*otated (FAIR) position.**

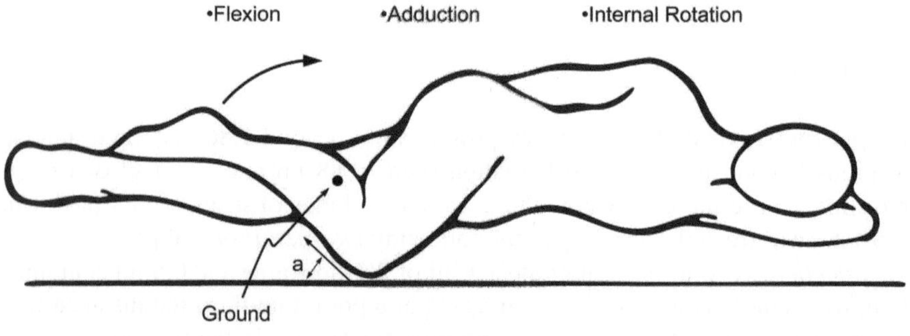

2. Ultrasound to piriformis muscle, while leg is placed in flexion, adduction, and internal rotation (FAIR): 2.25–2.5 watts/cm^2 for 10–14 min. *Beware* of patients with any hypoesthesia or anesthesia due to neurological or surgical causes in the dorsal lumbosacral region. *Beware* of cavitation in post-laminectomy patients.***
3. Wipe off ultrasound gel.
4. Hot packs or cold spray at the same location × 10 min.
5. Stretch the piriformis muscle for 10–14 min by applying manual pressure to the muscle's inferior border, being careful not to press downward, rather directing pressure tangentially, toward the ipsilateral shoulder.****

6. Myofascial release at lumbosacral paraspinal muscles.
7. McKenzie exercises.
8. Use a lumbosacral corset when post-surgical patients are placed in the FAIR position[2].*****

Duration: Two to three times weekly for 1–2 months (Table 7.1).

Table 7.1 Physical therapy protocol for piriformis syndrome

*Patients usually require 2–3 months of biweekly therapy for 60–70% improvement	**Because it is painful, patients often subtly shift to prone. This must be avoided because it works to place the affected leg in abduction, not adduction, greatly reducing the stretch placed on the piriformis muscle
***Cavitation is unreported in more than 20,000 treatments	****Unless explicitly stated, therapists may tend to knead or massage the muscle, which is useless or worse. The muscle must be stretched perpendicular to its fibers, in a plane that is tangent to the buttock at the point of intersection of the piriformis muscle and the sciatic nerve, but approximately three-fourth of an inch deep to the buttock (i.e., just below the gluteus maximus)
	*****In patients with previous lumbar laminectomy, a lumbosacral corset during PT may reduce the tendency toward hyperlordosis

John Stewart rightly criticized this treatment protocol for its non-specificity, pointing out that myofascial release of the lumbosacral paraspinal musculature and McKenzie exercises would be therapeutic for herniated disc as well. We did the myofascial release and McKenzie exercises to free up the anterior and posterior lumbar roots in order to give the lumbosacral plexus and origins of the sciatic nerve more slack, which would, in turn, enable the sciatic nerve to respond to the pressure of a tightened piriformis muscle by moving aside. Even before looking at the results, we may ask, would this criticism vitiate the significance of positive results?

We do not think so. These 918 patients had seen an average of 6.5 clinicians before coming to us, and in most cases had had at least one course of physical therapy directed toward the lumbar spine. The average FAIR-test positive (FTP) patient had sought relief for 6.2 years. It was impossible to trace this in each case, but in a subgroup of 440 patients, the ones for whom exhaustive records were available, 320 (73%) had undergone at least one negative lumbsacral MRI (and no positive ones) and 120 (27%) had at least one positive MRI. In fact these groups were quite similar in outcome, illustrating once again that one can have two diagnoses at the very same time. The piriformis diagnosis just happened to contribute more to their symptoms than the radiculopathy in these cases.

---

[2]In patients with previous lumbar laminectomy, a lumbosacral corset during PT may reduce the tendency toward hyperlordosis in these patients. It is a safety measure after fusion, scoliosis surgery, and disc replacement as well.

How Does Dual Diagnosis Affect Treatment?

Only two differences appeared between those with and those without positive MRIs. First, the 129 patients with positive MRI had, on the average, taken a full year longer to seek treatment for a second condition, the piriformis syndrome. The "diagnosis of exclusion" mentality might have contributed to their extra year of discomfort. Caregivers might have reasoned: "They have a herniated disc. Why search for other pathology [although they do not respond even to surgical intervention!]." At any rate they waited a full year more before looking further. Secondly, slightly more of the group which had both negative MRI and negative EMG improved 50% or more, on the average. There might possibly have been a minor contribution of pain from the untreated spinal diagnosis in the other cases (Table 7.2).

Table 7.2 Whether MRI were positive for spinal pathology or not, the treatment of injection and physical therapy for patients with positive FAIR tests was equally effective. The same held for the results of conventional electrodiagnostic studies

MRI of patients with positive fair test ($n = 449$)				
MRI	Number	Improved >50% (%)	Mean improvement (%)	Year of pain
Positive	129	74.7	62.3	6.9
Negative	320	74	61.5	5.8
Negative MRI and EMG	179	76	61.8	5.9

Of course we treated hamstring tears and ischial bursitides in our facilities, the people who did not seem to have piriformis syndrome, either by clinical criteria or by FAIR test. Most of them had sacroiliac joint derangement or far lateral disc herniations. Others had spondylolisthesis that was not thought to be clinically relevant or trochanteric bursitis. Naturally, the protocols for treating them were quite distinct and a function of their diagnoses and are not considered further here (see Table 7.3).

Tabulation of Results

Characteristics of Patients with Positive FAIR Tests

Follow-up after 6, 12, 24, 36, and 48 months: Follow-ups in person, by telephone or through the mail, sought answers to items in the same questionnaire used at the initial visit, along with the visual analog scale. Telephone interviews replaced the visual analog scale with the question, "What percentage, if any, have you improved or worsened since your first visit to our offices?" This question was also asked in each written questionnaire.

Table 7.3 Patients with positive FAIR tests responded more favorably to piriformis injection and physical therapy regardless of their signs and symptoms, suggesting that the test and the treatment were directed toward the same pathology, and that the functional test identifies piriformis syndrome more accurately than the set of signs and symptoms

Positive FAIR test improves success rates in patients with and without two of the three clinical characteristics of PS.

	Patients with two of three PS characteristics		Patients without two of three PS characteristics	
Outcome group	Surgery (n)	Conservative therapy (n)	Surgery (n)	Conservative Therapy (n)
50% Improvement	70.8%	84.1%	85.7%	68.3%
p-Value	(17/24)	(279/353)	(6/7)	(138/202)
Mean improvement (n)	60.2%	69.1%	77.1%	57.9%
	[24]	[353]	[7]	[202]
FAIR-test positive	80%	91.4%	66.7%	81.2%
50% improvement (n)	(28/35)	(381/417)	(2/3)	(69/85)
FAIR-test positive	66.7%	71.7%	50%	66.7%
Mean improvement (n)	[35]	[417]	[3]	[85]
FAIR-test negative	72.2%	82.1%	100%	57.8%
50% improvement (n)	(8/11)	(87/106)	(4/4)	(77/116)
FAIR-test negative	69.1%	57.1%	97.5%	50.9%
Mean improvement (n)	[11]	[106]	[4]	[116]

Results

Over 79% of patients meeting two or more of the clinical criteria for piriformis syndrome (279/353) improved by 50% or more (average improvement: 71%). FTP patients meeting two or more of the clinical criteria for piriformis syndrome showed 50% or greater improvement in 256 of 308 cases (83.1%). Of the 109 FTP patients meeting less than two clinical criteria, 82 (75.2%) improved by 50% or more (average: 57.9%). Only 30 of the 45 (67%) patients meeting fewer than two clinical criteria and having negative FAIR tests improved 50% or more (average: 52.5%). This is illustrated in Table 7.7. In follow-up, 308 of these patients reported their outcomes.

On average of 10.2 months' follow-up (SD = 11.7) after the conservative treatment ouitlined above, 79% of the people with positive FAIR tests who responded ($n = 665$) had achieved at least 50% improvement in their painful symptoms, and the 385 FAIR-test positive (FTP) responders showed a mean 62.8% reduction in disability related to their original complaints of low back, buttock, and/or sciatic pain. The FAIR-test negative responders improved 54.8% ($n = 209$), with a 54.8% reduction in related disability (Table 7.3). The FTP group of 665 patients had seen an average of 6.5 clinicians over the average 6.2 years since they had contracted piriformis syndrome. Their improvement was consistent regardless of whether their posterior tibial or peroneal branches were involved (see Table 7.4).

To date, we have been able closely to follow 46 FTP patients who either were unsatisfied with the results of conservative treatment or did not choose to undergo conservative therapy, who have gone to surgery, with 30 (65.2%) achieving 50% relief or more. Anatomic variations were reported in 6 of 46 cases (13.0%), approximating the percentage seen in cadaveric studies of the general population [6–8]. Reduction of sural sensory nerve action potential (more than 30% reduction) on the affected side was seen not more than 20% of the time in any group (Table 7.4).

Table 7.4 Surgical results may be negatively skewed since misdiagnosed patients would be more likely to fail conservative therapy

Characteristics of piriformis patients with positive FAIR tests*

Fair-test positive nerve	Improved 50% with conservative therapy (n)	Improved 50% with surgery (n)	Average number of clinicians seen (n)	Average number of years with pain (n)	Sural SNAP reduced 50% on affected side (n)
Posterior tibial nerve	79.19 [345]	21 [30]	6.5 [345]	6.6 [345]	1 [15]
Peroneal nerve	79.00 [320]	9 [16]	6.6 [320]	5.8 [320]	3 [15]
Total	79.098 [665]	30 [46]	6.55 [665]	6.2 [665]	4 [30]

*The nerve that had the most positive FAIR test was used when both nerves showed significant delay.

Leg-length discrepancy, contracted iliopsoas muscle, prolonged sitting, poor seating, and over-enthusiastic exercise can be countered with heel-lift, iliopsoas stretching and gait training, breaks in sitting, better chairs and vehicular seats, and cutting down on repetitive exercise programs, respectively.

We examined the conditions surrounding a positive FAIR test further. To determine whether other factors significantly influenced outcome, we evaluated 71 characteristics recorded in extensive interview and physical examination. The details are presented in Table 7.5. This table may be used to determine the clinical likelihood of piriformis syndrome in a given patient with his/her individual symptoms and signs. For example, 86.5% (283/337) of the patients with sciatica, buttock pain on flexion, adduction and internal rotation, tenderness in the region where the piriformis muscle intersects with the sciatic nerve, and greater pain when sitting versus standing had positive FAIR tests. *In toto*, 308 of these patients reported their longer term outcomes. With conservative therapy, 259 (84.1%) of them reported 50% or more improvement.

We have constructed a computable odds ratio table. One reason to consider this is its reliable prediction of success with conservative therapy. An automatic calculator is available on the Internet at *sciatica.org* for clinicians interested in using this tool.

But there is a second way in which this statistical correlation of other symptoms and signs is useful to us. By relating other aspects of these patients to the functionally-made electrodiagnosis, it may appear more reasonable that the prolongation of the H reflex through stretching the piriformis muscle across it actually

Table 7.5 These concomitants of piriformis syndrome may help clinicians recognize when to look for it, when it is present, and the odds of successful treatment

Characteristics favoring a successful outcome in treating piriformis syndrome according to this protocol

	p-Value	Odds ratio	95% CI
Positive fair test	<0.001	2.226	1.42–3.60
SLRM[a]	<0.001	2.83	1.69–4.73
Overuse	0.001	2.05	1.35–3.12
Tender piriformis	0.003	1.97	1.27–3.06
SLRM	0.007	2.03	1.22–3.06
Sitting worse than standing	0.007	1.77	1.17–2.68
Male gender	0.17	1.67	1.10–2.50
Illiotibial band syndrome	0.028	2.87	1.12–7.38
SLRM	0.32	3.83	1.12–13.06
Injection	0.03	1.55	1.05–2.31
Non-sciatic PSW	0.035	1	1.05–4.06
SLRM	0.013	3.29	1.25–8.42
L2 SLRM[b]	0.04	0.36[c]	0.13–0.95
Peroneal polyphasics	0.041	2.02	1.03–3.98
Non-sciatic polyphasics	0.041	2.51	1.04–6.06
SLRM	0.48	3	1.01–8.92
Clinical piriformis	<0.001	3.32	2.25–4.90
Years of pain	0.041	0.91	

Note: Values are from logistic model (univariate analyses) and stepwise regression; receiver operation characteristic (ROC) = 0.692 ($n = 651$ patients, 514 successful outcomes).
CI, confidence interval; PSW, positive sharp waves; SLRM, stepwise logistic regression model.
[a]ROC = 0.692.
[b]Either radiculopathy or positive electromyographic findings.
[c]Electromyographic abnormalities at L2 are associated with a lower probability of 50% improvement. They may imply a different origin for piriformis abnormalities. See text below.

is responsible for the lower extremity complaints. For example, a negative correlation of 50% improvement with ipsilateral L2 abnormalities suggests that iliopsoas weakness or dyscontrol is linked with piriformis hypertrophy or greater-than-normal contraction of that muscle, since both are external rotators of the thigh. The positive correlation between non-sciatic positive sharp waves and positive FAIR test just confirms what is abundantly clear already: that people can have more than one diagnosis, and one may actually raise the likelihood of another (Table 7.6).

Surgical Corroboration of the FAIR Test

We suggested surgery to those people who did not improve with conservative therapy, and sent them, as well as one individual who initially preferred surgery to conservative treatment, to the orthopedic surgeons most experienced in piriformis syndrome. Drs Christopher Mickelson of Columbia College of Physicians and

Table 7.6 The FAIR test appears to be helpful to patients with piriformis syndrome

Overall utility of the FAIR test			
	FAIR test		
	Positive	Negative	Chi square, degrees of freedom
Two or more PS criteria met			
50% Improvement	83.1% (256/309)	75.5% (77/102)	
p	0.12		2.44, 1 df
Mean improvement	70.6% [308]	63.3% [102]	
p	0.05		
Fewer than two PS criteria met			
50% Improvement	81.3% (52/64)	66.7% (30/45)	
p	0.13		2.88, 1 df
Mean improvement	66.7% [64]	52.5% [45]	
p	0.028		
All patients			
50% Improvement	82.8% (308/372)	74.8% (107/147)	
p	0.015		5.97, 1 df
Mean improvement	69.6% [372]	59.9% [147]	
p	0.003		

Surgeons, Bryan Kelly of Hospital for Special Surgery, and Jacob Rozbruch of Beth Israel Medical Center saw and did surgery on most of the 46 patients whom we were able to follow closely.

Generally the surgery was neurolysis of the sciatic nerve, in which adhesions from the muscle and the underlying ischiofemoral ligament to the nerve were cleared. But in approximately 15% of patients, where anomalous passage of the piriformis muscle by the sciatic nerve was seen, the muscle was excised. These results are consistent with the success rates seen in the patient group selected by FAIR-test positivity, but are perhaps even more impressive, since this surgery is about as specific as one could get to treating the piriformis syndrome without doing much to affect radiculopathic pain (Table 7.7).

Table 7.7 Characteristics and outcome of patients without piriformis versus those with piriformis according to conservative or surgical treatment

Improvement of piriformis, non-piriformis, and surgical patients				
	Weight (n)	Age (n)	Average months followup (n)	Percent of average improvement (n)
Piriformis conservative	150.99 [671]	54 [671]	10.2 [665]	79 [665]
Piriformis absent	149.57 [332]	57 [331]	9.9 [339]	55 [339]
Piriformis surgery	149.12 [46]	49 [46]	16 [46]	65 [46]

Surgery's efficacy may be underrated here since any misdiagnosed patients would have tended to fail physical therapy, and thus would be over-represented in the surgical series, reducing the surgeons' success rates below what a series of "naïve" surgical candidates with piriformis syndrome would be. The comparable success rates of surgical and non-surgical treatment suggest that the provocative maneuver of the FAIR test not only correctly identifies piriformis syndrome but also that this diagnostic entity was the main pain generator in nearly two-third of the surgical cases.

One surgical technique severs the piriformis muscle's connection to the conjoint tendon at the greater trochanter, attempting to relieve its pressure on the sciatic nerve with minimal trauma to the nerve itself. Without neural scanning, we caution against this technique because we have seen several patients with inferior gluteal arteries wrapped around the sciatic nerve, and others in which one or both branches of the nerve perforate the piriformis muscle. Both of these conditions would be missed and mistreated without neural scan or direct visualization.

In a previous paper [2], we cited a surgical series from Dr. Stephen Ringel, an orthopedic surgeon, done with Dr. Cheryl Weber, a physiatrist, both of Lubbock, Texas. The FAIR test was used to diagnose patients, and then repeated as soon as incision stability allowed. The H reflex + M wave (the H loop) had a mean delay of 2.25 ms in pre-operative FAIR testing and a delay of 1.28 ms in post-operative testing (Table 7.8).

We used the same functional diagnostic technique, the FAIR test, in two studies supported by Allergan and Elan, the companies that manufactured botulinum neurotoxins A and B, respectively, at the time of our studies. Each investigation was approved by the IRB at Sound Shore Medical Center in New Rochelle, New York.

Table 7.8 Changes are differences between pre- and post-surgical FAIR tests when both are present

Pre- and post-surgical FAIR tests					
Patient	Pre-op. test (ms)	Post-op. test (ms)	Test change (ms)	SD of change	Clinical outcome
1	NO	1.46	NO	NO	Excellent
2	2.29	1.04	1.25	2.0	Excellent
3	3.54	2.08	1.46	3.34	Excellent
4	0.83	0.00	0.83	1.34	Good
5	NO	1.25	NO		Excellent
6	2.08	NO	NO		Excellent
7	2.49	0.83	1.86	3.00	Excellent
8	NO	1.04	NO		Poor
Total	11.23	7.70	5.40	8.68	
Mean	2.25	1.28	1.35	2.17	

The average change was 2.17 SD. (SD as found in our study [4]).
NO, not obtained.

The study with botulinum neurotoxin A used the same parameters for diagnosis, and the same basic location for injection, and the same physical therapy. It came up with essentially the same success-rate, though 50% improvement was seen within 2–3 weeks, versus 2–3 months seen in the 1,014 patient study using steroid and lidocaine injections [2].

In the second study, a dose-finding investigation using botulinum neurotoxin B (Bt-B), we again used the same diagnostic criteria and technique, and the same physical therapeutic regimen, but we changed the exclusion criteria and the injection protocol [3, 8].

Exclusion criteria included previous exposure to botulinum neurotoxins, electrophysiologic evidence of paraspinal denervation or denervation of pelvic or lower limb muscles not innervated by the sciatic nerve, and pregnancy.

There were three changes in the injection protocol. First, since this was a dose-finding study, we divided 32 FTP patients into four equal groups, injecting 5,000, 7,500, 10,000, and 12,500 units of Bt-B into each patient of successive groups. We approximated these doses as 150, 200, 250, and 300 IU of botulinum neurotoxin type A, respectively.

Secondly, we used an EMG injectible needle in order to be certain that we were injecting into the piriformis muscle. Third, we injected one-fourth the total of each dose into four separate locations in the piriformis muscle. Since botulinum neurotoxins have their effect at the myoneural junction, we reasoned that injecting them into different sites would maximally weaken the muscle's grip on the sciatic nerve. How could we be sure we were actually doing so? (Fig. 7.2)

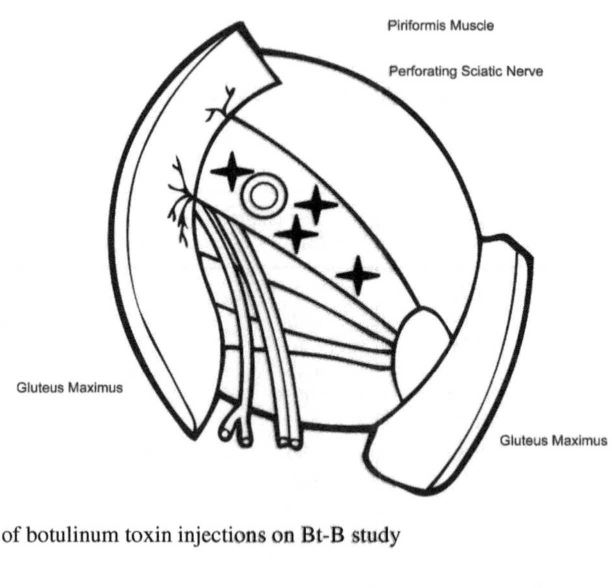

Fig. 7.2 Sites of botulinum toxin injections on Bt-B study

Locating the Piriformis Muscle

The chief difficulty was distinguishing the piriformis muscle from the gluteus maximus that lies directly above it. To solve this problem, we began with the patient in the FAIR position, inserting an EMG-injectible needle approximately 5/8 of an inch, then asking the patient to abduct the flexed thigh. If we saw no interference pattern, we advanced the needle one-fourth inch and tried again. Once we obtained a good interference pattern, we took it that the needle tip was in either the gluteus maximus or the piriformis muscle. At that point we asked the patient to compress his or her thighs together and extend the hip. If we saw an interference pattern at that point, we took it that the needle was in the gluteus maximus and advanced the needle further. Then we asked the patient to abduct the flexed thigh again, to confirm that the needle was still in either the gluteus maximus or piriformis. Given a confirmatory interference pattern, we then asked the patient to extend the thigh again. *Not* seeing an interference pattern at that point was evidence that we were *not* in the gluteus maximus, and so we injected the botulinum neurotoxin. We reasoned that because there was an interference pattern seen on abduction, the needle was either in the gluteus maximus maximus or the piriformis muscle, and since there was no interference pattern on hip extension, it was not in the gluteus maximus. Logically speaking, it was an instance of A or B and not B: therefore A. Therefore, we believed we were injecting into the piriformis muscle.

This maneuver itself may be seen as an instance of functional EMG used for injection.

The 32 patients had average age of 53 years, with a mean 6.2 years of sciatica. They had seen an average of 5.8 clinicians before entering the study. Two patients left the study, each because MRIs ordered in our offices turned up large herniated intervertebral discs in the lumbar spine for which they subsequently had surgical procedures. Both were replaced by patients from the waiting-list.

Clinical improvement by the visual analog scale was greatest at 12,500 units of Bt-B (overall analysis of variance, p = 0.013) (see Table 7.9). All groups had their most dramatic improvement between weeks 2 and 5, when the common adverse

Table 7.9 The highest dose of botulinum neurotoxin B brought about the most dramatic reduction in pain at weeks 2 and 4

Comparison of VAS changes at different doses of BT-B

Different dose groups (units)	2 Weeks [Mean ± SE (n)]	4 Weeks [Mean ± SE (n)]	8 Weeks [Mean ± SE (n)]	12 Weeks [Mean ± SE (n)]	Overall [Mean ± SE (n)]
5,000	−2.6±0.28 (8)	−2.4±0.78 (8)	−2.4±0.75 (8)	−3.4±0.89 (8)	−2.61±0.59 (8)
7,500	−2.14±1.14 (7)	−2.83±0.78 (6)	−3.2±1.19 (5)	−1.3±0.87 (7)	−2.12±0.75 (7)
10,000	−2.5±0.51 (6)	−2.56±0.92 (6)	−4.16±1.08 (5)	−2.62±1.14 (4)	−2.89±0.60 (6)
12,000	−5.55±0.55 (5)	−5.39±0.86 (5)	−3.60±1.62 (5)	−3.0±0.74 (4)	−4.51±0.30 (5)

effects of dry mouth and dysphagia were also most evident. Both the improvement and the side effects showed a dose-related response curve (Table 7.9).

FAIR test values closely paralleled clinical improvement. Correlation of the posterior tibial FAIR test and the visual analog scale had a sensitivity of 72% and a specificity of 77% ($\chi^2 = 17.02$; $p < 0.0001$). This relationship yields independent verification of the efficacy of treatment focused closely on the piriformis muscle. The closely parallel, almost tandem variation of patient relief and side effects further suggests that the medication injected into the piriformis muscle was the cause of both. This study brought out an intimate connection between patient symptoms and the FAIR-test values, something one would see if the test actually recorded the pathogenetic mechanism. The covariance of side effects and main effect, and of the visual analog scale and the FAIR test, suggests that compression by the piriformis muscle, as measured by the functional H-reflex comparison of the FAIR test, is the actual cause of the patients' symptoms, and is specifically treated by the injection (Fig. 7.3; Table 7.10).

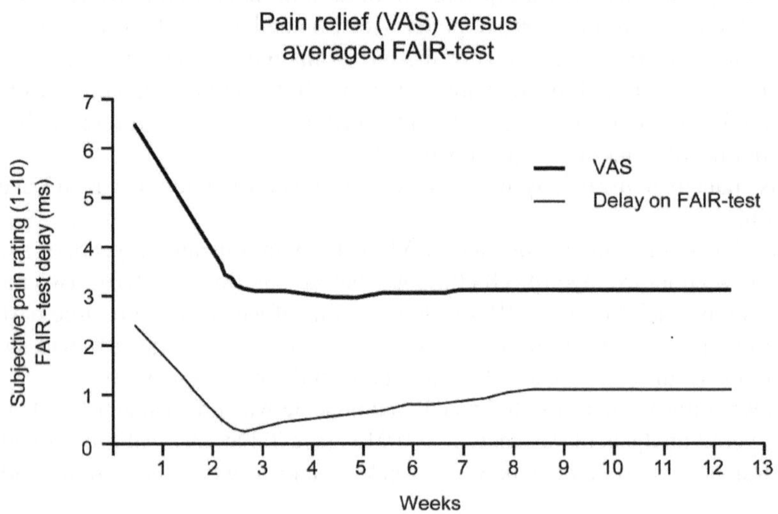

Fig. 7.3 Parallel course of pain and delay in FAIR test

Summary

Contemporary work indicates that piriformis syndrome is a common and remediable cause of sciatica, with a family of symptom- and sign-set that overlaps the symptoms and signs that are also associated with herniated nucleus pulposis, spinal stenosis, and arthritic narrowing of neuroforamina, but which can be distinguished from them through careful history and physical, functional electrophysiological diagnosis, and MRI, including neural scanning. According to some studies, piriformis syndrome appears to be among the most common of these diagnoses [9].

Table 7.10 Prolongation of H-reflex latency in FAIR position versus sciatica and buttock pain—Bt-B study

VAS parallels FAIR-test delay

	FAIR test		
VAS	>1.86 ms	<1.86 ms	Total
>5	26	10	36
<5	10	33	43
Total	36	43	79

Coefficient of correlation = 0.77
$\chi^2 = 17.02$
$p<0.0001$; df = 1

In Chapter 6, we showed the diagnostic methodology, with correlation to the symptoms that would identify the piriformis syndrome. In this chapter, we have given evidence that the syndrome so identified admits of successful treatment through conservative and surgical means that focus on the piriformis muscle. We must now turn to a third example of functional EMG.

References

1. Stewart, JD. "The piriformis syndrome is overdiagnosed." *Muscle Nerve.* 2003 Nov;28(5): 644–6.
2. Fishman, LM, Dombi, GW, Michaelsen, C, Ringel, SV, Rosbruch, J, Rosner, B, Weber, C. "Piriformis Syndrome: Diagnosis, treatment and outcome- a ten year study." *Arch Phys Med Rehabil.* 2002;83(3):295–302.
3. Fishman, LM, Anderson, C, Rosner, B. "Botulinum toxin type A and physical therapy in the treatment of piriformis syndrome." *Am J Phys Med Rehabi.* 2002 Dec;81(12):936–42.
4. Fishman, LM, Konnoth, C, Rozner, B. "Botulinum neurotoxin type B and physical therapy in the treatment of piriformis syndrome: a dose-finding study." *Am J Phys Med Rehabil.* 2004;83:42–50.
5. Fishman, LM, Konnoth, C, Rosner, B "EMG and Botulinum neurotoxin type B in the diagnosis and treatment of thoracic outlet syndrome." *Am J Phys Med Rehabil.* 2004 Mar;83(3):p. 228 (abstract).
6. Yeoman, W "Relation of arthritis of sacro-iliac joint to sciatica." Lancet. 1928;1119–22.
7. Pecina, M "Contribution to the etiological explanation of the piriformis syndrome." *Acta Anat.* 1979;105:181–7.
8. Gotlin, R "Clinical correlation of an anatomical investigation into piriformis syndrome *Proc NY Soc Phys Med Rehabil.* 1991;24(6):11.
9. Filler, AG, Haynes, J, Jordan, SE, Prager, J, Villablanca, P, Farahani, K, McBride, DQ, Tsuruda, JS, Morisoli, B, Batzdorf, U, Johnson, JP "Sciatica of nondisc origin and piriformis syndrome:diagnosis by magnetic resonance neurography and interventional magnetic resonance imaging with outcome study of resulting treatment." *J Neurosurg Spine.* 2005;2:99–115.

Chapter 8
Radiculopathy vs. Spinal Stenosis: Evocative Electrodiagnosis Identifies the Main Pain Generator

Abstract Cadaveric studies measuring up to 63% narrowing of the stenotic spine with extension suggests that intraspinal conductions in the cauda equina might be delayed by extension. In this chapter, we examine delays in H-reflexes brought about by extension and then use this delay as an estimate of the clinical significance of patients' stenosis. This is useful in determining how great a factor the stenosis is when it is accompanied by a herniated disc, for it helps clinicians decide which of two conditions should be the chief focus of therapy.

Keywords Foraminal stenosis · Latency · Gaenslen's sign · Positionally exacerbated spinal stenosis (PESS) · Jendrassik maneuver

Intraspinal Stenosis vs. Foraminal Stenosis

In the case of thoracic outlet syndrome and piriformis syndrome, we were searching for some objective way to identify what had previously been "diagnoses of exclusion," entities that were mainly sought when no other diagnosis could be found. We worked to find an electrophysiological test that affirmed these diagnoses and attempted more precisely to characterize conditions that had only vaguer connotation. After doing so, we had to be sure that the tests supporting these characterizations led to effective treatment.

In the current chapter, we discuss another electrophysiological test, but this time it will act as a decision procedure to determine which of two well-established conditions makes the greater contribution to the symptoms of a patient that has them both. In this situation, the diagnoses each have effective treatments. But although the conditions may coexist, the treatments are incompatible!

This is needed when a patient's symptoms may be explained by two different diagnoses both of which have been confirmed, but where the two diagnoses have dissimilar treatments. That situation frequently involves a herniated disc and associated spinal stenosis. It is not rare to have these two diagnoses joined by spondylolisthesis, either. The unfortunate part is that from a therapeutic point of view, they are opposites. Spinal stenosis and spondylolisthesis are best treated in flexion, and are worsened by extension, while herniated nucleus pulposis is more likely to respond

L.M. Fishman, A.N. Wilkins, *Functional Electromyography*,
DOI 10.1007/978-1-60761-020-5_8,

to extension, and its symptoms are generally exacerbated by flexion. Since the two occur together in a fair number of cases, the therapeutic community frequently faces the options of either treating one condition while exacerbating the other or doing nothing at all. These unpleasant alternatives can only be avoided by determining which of the two conditions is the main pain generator, and therefore the primary one to treat.

But we may, with functional EMG, take advantage of the different neuroskeletal changes that take place with flexion and extension. We may view electrophysiological changes as reflecting clinical and neurological repercussions of the structural changes that positional variations produce in herniated spinal discs and stenosis. Since the course of the H reflex traverses the entire lumbar spine, and is replicable under normal conditions, it is a fair vehicle to carry these changes. The idea is to determine the changes in the H reflex from flexion and extension, as compared to the anatomical condition. This may not be too far-fetched, since extension has been noted to further narrow the stenotic intraspinal canal by up to 63% [1–5], while the herniated portion of a lumbar discs described by McKenzie and others to retract during extension, further opening neuroforamina [6].

As we reasoned earlier, if electrophysiological investigations are extensions of the physical examination, then provocative maneuvers such as extension and flexion might well have electrodiagnostic correlates. Our task here was to find the conditions in which we could reliably evoke them.

Some maneuvers are not always provocative. Terming something "provocative" insinuates that its effects are more or less unpleasant, while some maneuvers, such as the Jendrassic maneuver, enhance normal response; it might be better to call this type of maneuver "evocative." As a case in point, extension may reduce neuroforaminal narrowing in herniated intervertebral disc, reducing pain, and shortening the H-reflex latency. Thus lumbar spinal extension might be *provocative* for spinal stenosis, causing discomfort and sensory symptoms, but *evocative*, and actually improve these same symptoms in foraminal disease due to disc herniation. Extension may reduce H-reflex latency and enhance its amplitude, making visible a previously undetectable response. But although extension may be an evocative maneuver in neuroforaminal narrowing due to a soft tissue impingement, flexion may be provocative in the same situation and worsen conduction. For spinal stenosis, flexion may evoke a previously absent H reflex and F wave, or enhance the amplitude or diminish the latency of a pre-existing one, while extension may provoke just the reverse.

These opposite responses to the same maneuver are sometimes helpful for clinician in the situations we are about to encounter.

Strategies and Methods

We used a tripartite strategy. First we had to follow an exclusion-like preliminary phase, in which we identified people who had neither radiological nor electrophysiological problems apart from mild, moderate, or severe lumbar stenosis. To determine if there were a significant effect brought about by extension, we compared the H-reflex latency in the anatomical position to what we saw in extreme and prolonged extension. In the early phase, it seemed wise and compassionate to titrate sensitivity and specificity of the test vs. patient discomfort. Some of the initial candidates for the test did not qualify because they were unable to extend their spines at all. In other cases, extension was limited either by joint mobility or the by the pain that extension engendered. Although both these maneuvers (the anatomical positions of flexion and extension) and EMG are standard medical procedures of physicians and physical therapists, and are applied to patients with the general condition of lower back pain, patient consent was always obtained in this investigational phase (Fig. 8.1).

The relevant independent variables appeared to be as follows:

1. How much extension?
2. For how long

We found 13 patients with MRIs positive for some degree of spinal stenosis, but MRI and EMG negative for any foraminal pathology, and compared H reflex recorded just previously in the anatomical position with H-reflex latency every half-minute during 3 min in extension. We always examined the more symptomatic leg. If both legs were relatively equally involved on EMG and with regard to pain, strength and sensory function on clinical examination, then both legs were tested in both positions. In each case, H reflex latencies were elicited in the anatomical position and compared with H-reflex latencies in 3-min extension. Submaximal stimuli were applied at 0.1 ms, with the cathode proximal to avoid anodal block. Stimulus intensity was manipulated to find the maximal H-reflex amplitude, which had to be larger than the M response that preceded it. Stimuli were separated by 30 s. The latency was measured as the first departure from the isoelectric line. Where the onset was unclear, the positive or negative peak was taken to determine the variation between the responses in the anatomical and extended position (see Figs. 8.2 and 8.3).

Using filters at 100 and 10,000 Hz, setting time intervals and amplification at 5/500 ms divisions, and stimulating at a maximum of 0 32 mA, we found an average of 1.9 ms prolongation of the H reflex with 3-min extension, as compared with the H reflexes elicited in the anatomical position. The standard deviation for side-to-side variation in H-reflex latency is considered 0.5 ms [7]. We reasoned that the variation in H-reflex latency between one leg and another was likely to be equal to or greater than the difference between one leg and itself; therefore, this discrepancy of 1.9 ms was more than 3 and nearly 4 standard deviations beyond the mean for leg-to-itself variation, i.e., the intrinsic margin of error in measurement (Table 8.1).

The provocative maneuver appeared to register a significant change in the H reflex. There was a mean 1.9-ms delay, generally in the posterior tibial H-reflex latency, after 3 min of extension. The H reflex was studied in the limb(s) that on history, physical, and conventional NCV were the most involved. That might have been the most painful limb, the one with the denser sensory deficit, the one with

Fig. 8.1 Stenosis is evident in same-cut Fonar images of a normal lumbar spine in anatomical and extended positions

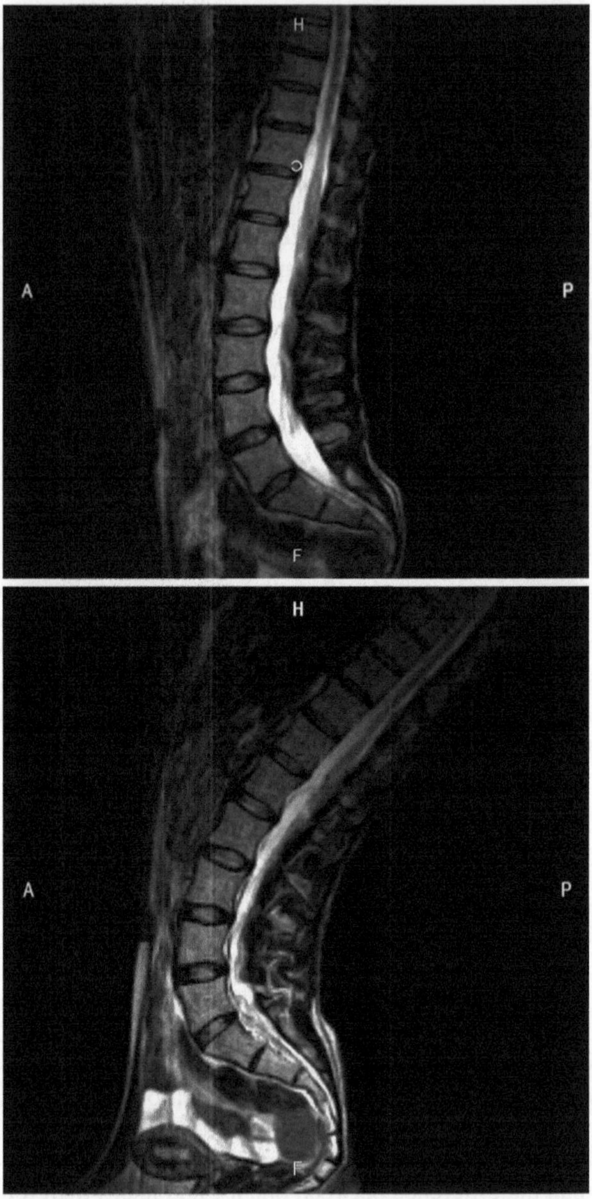

the most severe motor changes, or the one with the greatest H-reflex latency in the anatomical position. But even though these differences popped up, it was still possible that a number of other conditions would produce the same dynamic result. Delay in H reflexes with extension could reflect other conditions as well as stenosis, just as delay in median distal motor latency might be due to neuropathy as well as carpal tunnel syndrome.

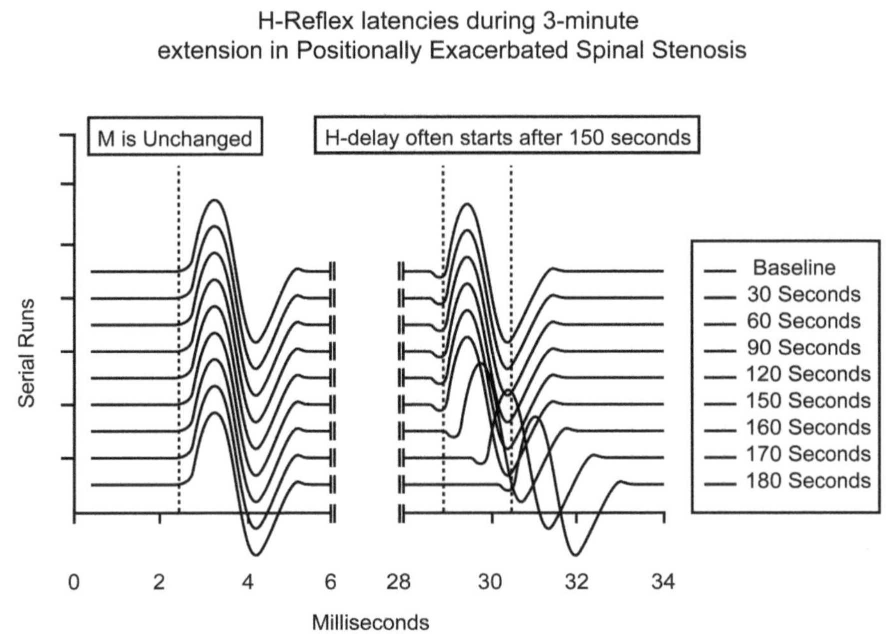

Fig. 8.2 The latencies of normal H reflexes with markers at first deviation from the isoelectric line may change when the patient is placed in extension. This maneuver can replicably delay the H reflex in less than 3 min. When the onset of either the anatomical or the extended H reflex is unclear, maxima and minima may be used in the comparison. In fact, being a summary of the entire muscle's depolarization that occurs in the reflex, a negative or positive peak may be more representative of the total reflex, and more replicable, than the first deviation from the isoelectric line in functional comparisons such as these

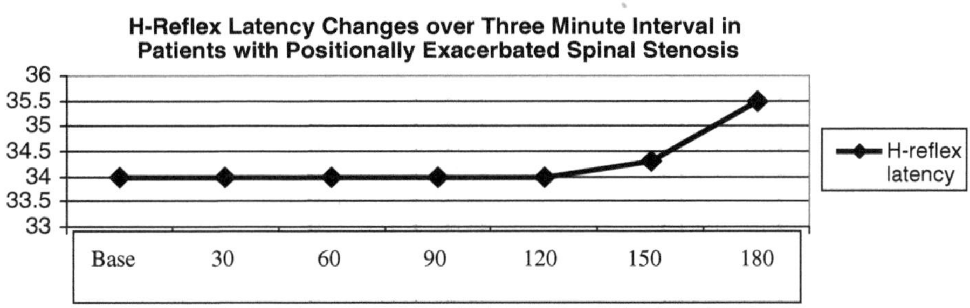

Fig. 8.3 Characteristic course of the H-reflex latencies taken every 30 s in patient with positionally exacerbated lumbar spinal stenosis during 3-min extension. It typically resembles an exponential rise in the last 20–30 s

This brought us to the second part of the strategy. At this point it was desirable to expand the study to other diagnoses which an electrodiagnostician would be considering under the same clinical conditions. In other words, we were then attempting to find a number of conditions under which extension had no effect on H-reflex latency.

Table 8.1 Delay of H reflex after 3 min maximal extension in patients with MRI-documented lumbar spinal stenosis

Patient	Gender	Age	MRI	EMG	Anatomical	3-min extension	Contralateral	Comments
1	F	41	Severe central and left lateral recess stenosis	Denervation left L5-S1-S2	28.4	31.3	23.7	Left posterior tibialis H reflex used
2	F	70	Stenosis	Denervation S1-2	37.1	39.4	Absent	Increased pain with extension
3	M	80	Stenosis	Denervation S1-2	33.74	34.1	34.9	LBP, hip and buttock pain
4	M	72	Stenosis	Normal	43	44.6	41.8	LBP
5	F	79	Stenosis L3-4 by CT	Bilateral L3-4-5-S1, chiefly 3-4	35.9	39.6	35.9	LBP
6	F	40	Stenosis	L L4-5-S1; R L5	35.1	36.7	32.5	Pain increased with walking
7	F	76	Stenosis S/P surgery	Normal	41.7	43.8		LBP
8	F	45	Mild/moderate L3-4 stenosis	2.1 ms delay in FAIR position	36.81	37.9	34.2	Bilateral electric shocks with heel strike and continuous bilateral sciatica
9	M	80	Stenosis; three surgeries	Bilateral L4-5	37.6	39.7	37	LBP, numbness left dorsal foot, lateral calf
10	F	54	Stenosis	Bilateral L5-S1, left posterior tibialis	34.3	37.4	34.7	LBP
11	F	44	Grade I spondylolisthesis stenosis; became grade II in 7 months	Normal at first, 7 months later bilateral denervation L5-S1	32.4	32.9	33	LBP left more than right, eventually had surgery
12	F	62	Stenosis	Normal	39.6	41.1	34.7	Lumbar eburnation and pain with extension
13	M	53	Stenosis	Vastus medialis, gastrocnemius, anterior tibialis	34.7	36.6	35	Left sciatica, foot drop
Totals	Four males	61.2			36.2	38.1	35.4	
Standard deviation		15.7			3.9	3.9	2.6	

It would be especially worthwhile to show that common causes of lower back pain and sciatica did *not* lead to any delay in H reflexes after 3-min extension. If there were such conditions, then the 3-min extension test could be used to distinguish between them and lumbar spinal stenosis.

To some extent clinical medicine is guided by suspicions. In the course of the last few years, we have tested a number of people whom we suspected had lumbar spinal stenosis, whom we already knew had herniated discs, piriformis syndrome, severe lumbar degenerative joint disease, sacroiliac derangement, or other musculoskeletal pathology.

These other conditions were capable of causing lower back pain and/or sciatica. Radiculopathy, arthritis, piriformis syndrome, and musculoskeletal pathology such as facet syndrome and sacroiliac joint derangement were the most common and therefore the most important "diagnoses for exclusion" here. For, if extension caused increased H-reflex latency in any of these diagnoses, it would sharply limit the utility of the 3-min extension test.

In fact, none of them seemed to be affected very much by 3 min in extension. We tested a number of patients who turned out to have "pure" lower lumbar radiculopathies, where subsequent MRIs showed no signs of spinal stenosis, a number of patients with significant radiculopathy-causing arthritic narrowing of neuroforamina at L4-5 and L5-S1 which turned out to be their only pathological findings, 10 patients with piriformis syndrome, again with normal MRIs, patients with normal MRIs apart from quite substantial facet arthritis, and another fairly substantial group that displayed positive Gaenslen signs, asymmetrical movement of the posterior superior iliac spines, and tenderness at the sacroiliac joints, but without neurological abnormalities. In this group also there was sufficient suspicion to order what later turned out to be totally normal MRIs and normal EMGs.

Apart from one patient with piriformis syndrome, who had a 1.4 ms delay in the posterior tibial H reflex after 3-min extension, none of the others showed a significant delay. These people showed no delay in their H-reflex latencies after 3-min extension. Patients with piriformis syndrome, radiculopathy, arthritis, and sacroiliac joint derangement were equally unresponsive to this evocative test.

Spondylolisthesis

In patients with spondylolisthesis, it was more complicated. This dynamic situation is what functional electrodiagnostics should handle best. The question for each patient with spondylosisthesis is whether extension causes enough anterior–posterior movement of the vertebrae to induce spinal stenosis, and whether that stenosis has clinical consequences. This might be a patient who has more pain standing and walking than sitting or lying down, for example. We found a number of cases of spondylolisthesis in which extension was painful, and in which there was no other cause than spondylolisthesis found on MRI for the patients' neurological

Table 8.2 Comparison of H reflexes in the anatomical position and after 3-min extension in patients with radiologically documented anterolisthesis Grades I and II, without other imaged pathology

Patient	Age	Spondylolisthesis on MRI	EMG	Anatomical	3 min	Contralateral
1	83	Spondylolisthesis L4-5	BL4-5-S1	34.8	36.8	32.53
2	54	Spondylolisthesis L5-S1	R H-reflex	34.3	37.7	34.7
3	44	Grade II spondylosisthesis L5-S1	BL5-S1	32.4	32.9	33
4	53	Grade II spondylolisthesis L5-S1	L L5-S1	31.7	33.4	32
5	62	Spondylolisthesis L3-4	N/A	33.6	36.8	33.8
6	73	Antero. L5-S1, retro L4-5	LL4-5; BL5-S1	34.5	35.8	28.6
7	82	Antero L5-S1, retro L4-5	RL5	34.5	37.8	35.9
8	68	Spondylolisthesis L5-S1	L L5, gastroc-nemius	39.4	40.7	37.71
9	71	Spondylosisthesis L3-4-5	BL5	35.5	37.3	32.7
10	68	Spondylolisthesis L4-5	BL4-5-S1	30	32.8	Absent
11	62	Spondylolisthesis L4-5	normal	39.6	41.1	34.7
12	60	Spondylolisthesis L4-5	normal	33.51	37.7	34.8
13	82	Grade II L4-5, Grade I L5-S1	BL5-S1	31.6	32.3	33
14	59	Spondylolisthesis L3-4	normal	34.7	37.87	34.3
Mean	65.78			34.29	36.50	33.67
SD	11.76			2.68	2.78	2.17

symptoms and signs. We then did the 3-min extension test for each of these patients (Table 8.2).

It appeared that at least some cases of anterolisthesis were capable of causing pain and other symptoms and signs through positionally exacerbated spinal stenosis, and that this evocative maneuver was able to pick up and quantify it. Most of these people did complain of pain, paraesthesias, and numbness that were worsened in positions of extension, e.g., looking at pictures at a museum.

We took the mean difference in H-reflex latencies at rest and after 3 min in extension that we had recorded in individuals who had conditions that were *not* affected by extension, and we used them as controls. The individuals with disc-related neuroforaminal narrowing actually showed a slight tendency toward reduction in H-reflex latencies after 3-min extension, but it did not reach statistical significance. Such a measurement might be significant in a sub-group of foraminal radiculopathies, but it was neither our purpose nor our good luck to find them in the course of this investigation.

Instead, the relative normalcy, the absence of any notable prolongation in the H-reflex latencies in people with other pathology but *not* spinal stenosis or spondylolisthesis gave us a powerful decision procedure: the fact that we found a significant delay in the people who had MRI-diagnosed spinal stenosis or spondylolisthesis but not in other related and frequently coexisting pathology suggested that the 3-min extension test might help us in cases of dual diagnosis to determine which of the two was contributing most to the patient's pain and disability.

We did not attempt to find correspondence between the severity of the stenosis and the size of the delay brought on by extension. There are several reasons that made us reluctant even to look. Firstly, the amount of extension was often limited by extraneous factors, such as arthritis, stiff muscles, and patient upper extremity strength. Secondly, the 3 min of our examination was entirely arbitrary, apart from there being reasonable time limits on any provocative or evocative test! Finally, although all patients had symptoms, some were brought about by standing, others by lying down, and some intermittently. Still others had symptoms that were present all the time. We were artificially, and under quite narrowly defined conditions, testing for electrophysiological changes that might or might not have been brought about maximally in the way we were testing.

Certainly there was a sharp contrast between the responses of people with spinal stenosis and other people, but it was more to the point of clinical usefulness that the contrast was just as unambiguous between patients with spinal stenosis and those with piriformis syndrome, herniated discs or other causes of foraminal stenosis such as severe spinal arthritis.

Is This Information Useful?

Now for the third part of the undertaking, the application of this relative litmus test. It is frequently desirable, and often quite difficult to determine which of two or more conditions is causing the lion's share of a patient's pain. Just as internists may wonder whether it is a patient's pneumonia or her urinary tract infection that is causing the fever, those who work in back pain have a dilemma when it comes to herniated discs and other conditions that also narrow the central canal. As luck would have it, there is not infrequently a corresponding spondylolisthesis, often at the same level as the herniated disc and the spinal stenosis. This is one situation in which the functional 3-min extension test appears to have value.

Over the past 2 years, we have encountered many patients posing exactly this dilemma. Subjecting them to the 3-min extension test has given us at first a hint, and as the statistics mounted, a clue turned into actual clinical guidance in how to treat them. It is well-documented, as we have said, that extension is helpful in disc-related radiculopathies, but harmful in spinal stenosis, while flexion is frequently beneficial in spinal stenosis, yet may exacerbate a herniation. Therefore, the test was not only valuable for the individual patient; but also viewing a number of outcomes in therapy guided by this procedure gave insight into the test's clinical utility.

In spondylolisthesis and spinal stenosis, we encounter this problem more than elsewhere: very often there is a herniated disc associated with spondylolisthesis, or causing stenosis, and at the same level. In this case conventional electrodiagnostic techniques would help us neither to identify which of these were the problem nor how much each condition contributed to a given patient's pain if they were both pain-generating. The pattern of denervation might be due to either condition. Yet the treatment for a stenotic central canal would be pretty much the opposite of what we would do for a radiculopathic neuroforaminal narrowing.

Probably there would be some cases where extension would cause stenosis and others in which it would not. Possibly, if the disc were responsible for the majority of the patient's symptoms, then the H-reflex latency would even shorten in extension due to a McKenzie-type effect. Could the 3-min extension test distinguish which condition(s) caused the problem?

In order to get a handle on this, we reviewed our testing of a fair number of people with sciatic symptoms and herniated disc as well as spondylolisthesis and/or spinal stenosis. The spondylolisthesis was generally at L4-5 or L5-S1, and generally grades I or II, as in Table 8.2 above. We then treated them according to the outcome of the 3-min extension test: those who showed delay with extension were treated with flexion exercises and the manual therapy for spinal stenosis, whether structural or the result of spondylolisthesis. The patients with herniated disc as well as structural stenosis or spondylolisthesis whose H reflexes were not prolonged significantly during 3 min of extension were treated with extension for herniated disc, in the manner of McKenzie [6] (Table 8.3).

Outcome of treatment assigned on the basis of delay or non-delay.

We believe these results are satisfactory, that the outcomes support using the 3-min test as a decision procedure in difficult cases such as these. Most of the patients who had significant delay of their H reflexes in the 3-min test, and were treated for spinal stenosis, appeared to improve quite a bit. Most of the patients whose H reflexes did not change significantly with extension, and were treated for foraminal stenosis, also did well (Tables 8.4, 8.5, and 8.6).

The outcomes seem to confirm the test's value, but to validate it in a rigorous way would require contrasting these outcomes with a randomly selected, matched control group treated without the test's guidance, or randomly assigned the flexion or extension protocols. There would be many confounding variables here, such as relative degrees of arthritis, activity levels, and therapist efficacy. Such a study might require quite a large sample size.

Discussion of the Procedure

1. Other factors that might change the H reflex with extension are as follows:

   A. Tension, such as the Jendrasik maneuver or the abdominal muscular stretching intrinsic to the 3-min test is known to influence the H reflex [8–11], but we saw neither an increase in H-reflex amplitude nor reduction in latency

Table 8.3 The 3-min extension test used to identify pain generators in the presence of both neuroforaminal stenosis and central canal stenosis and/or spondylolisthesis

Decision: spondylolisthesis and/or stenosis and HNP													
Name	Age	MRI	EMG	Comments	Anatomical	3 min	Difference	Other Side	3 min	Therapy	Outcome	Comments	Side
Positive													
1	56	Stenosis, radiculopathy, spondylolisthesis, all at L4-5	Denervation L4-5		29.7	30.7	1	39.4		For piriformis, then for central spinal stenosis	Stenosis treatment (flexion, manual therapy) eliminated LBP and left buttock pain. Right buttock pain continued	Probable successful spinal stenosis treatment	R
2	73	HNP and stenosis	Denervation left L4-5		35.9	38.1	2.2	34.8		Flexion, manual therapy	Good	Also piriformis syndrome	R
3	69	HNP L2-S1; severe neuroforaminal narrowing and stenosis L4-5-S1	Bilateral L4-5; left L5-S1	Bilateral LBP, left sciatica	34.9	36.7	1.8	34.9		PT, flexion	Considerably improved	Had 13 sessions	L
4	40	Stenosis, status post fusion	Denervation at incision site	Severe intermittent pain along incision site: L2-S2	35.1	36.7	1.6	32.5		Flexion, manual therapy	75–85% in 3 weeks	Severe abdominal pain, low B12	L

Table 8.3 (continued)

Decision: spondylolisthesis and/or stenosis and HNP

Name	Age	MRI	EMG	Comments	Anatomical	3 min	Difference	Other Side	3 min	Therapy	Outcome	Comments	Side
5	80	Significant stenosis L3-4 and HNP with moderate stenosis L4-5 and L5-S1	L3-4 L	Severe bilateral sciatica, LBP worsened with extension	40	43.7	3.7	41.9	44.5	Core strengthening	Temporary, slight	Received wrong therapy at first. Subsequently had 50% improvement with three epidural injections, sought surgical consultation	B
6	72	Grade I spondylolisthesis at the L2-3 and L4-5, mild/moderate spinal stenosis; HNP right L5-S1 compressing thecal sacs bilaterally and centrally	Bilateral denervation L4-5-S1		29.6	31.1	1.5	29.2		PT: flexion, manual therapy	50% improvement	Used peroneal H reflex	R
7	49	Moderate/severe stenosis L4-5 and bilateral foraminal narrowing L4-5-S1	Bilateral denervation L4-5-S1; bilateral H-reflex delay with flexion, adduction, internal rotation	Bilateral sciatica for 2 years, ascending bipedal numbness worsened by walking	37.8	39.7	1.9	38.8		Subsequently had fusion laminectomy, now 100% painless	???	History of piriformis syndrome that was successfully treated 5 years before.	L

Table 8.3 (continued)

Decision: spondylolisthesis and/or stenosis and HNP

Name	Age	MRI	EMG	Comments	Anatomical	3 min	Difference	Other Side	3 min	Therapy	Outcome	Comments	Side
8	67	Spondylolisthesis L3-4-5, HNP L2-3	Slight denervation left L5-S1	History of piriformis syndrome	46.4	49.1	2.7	42.2		Flexion exercises	90% improvement in seven sessions		L
9	60	Central HNP L5-S1 narrowing central canal and right neuroforamen	Denervation L5-S1,S3	Abrupt incontinence, penile sensory changes	28.3	31.4	3.1	26.3	27.7	Sent to ER			L
Mean	62.71				38.18	37.47	−0.71	35.56					
SD	12.771496			SD	5.48	6.16		5.55					
Negative													
10	48	HNP and spondylosisthesis L2-3	Bilateral denervation S1-S4	Vaginal and anal causalgia, coccygeal pain	31.8	31.8	0	33.2	33.2	PT	Anal and coccygeal pain relieved 100%; coccygeal pain unchanged	Pain mainly central	R
11	67	Stenosis L 3-4, HNP left L2-3 and right L4-5, scoliosis	Denervation right L4-5, left L5-S1, delayed left H reflexes	Degenerative scoliosis, "cottony" feeling at both feet	30.4	30.4	0	31.5	31.5	One session	Advised referring chiropractor to do McKenzie-type work	100% improved in 1 month	L
12	74	Severe stenosis and severe neuroforaminal narrowing L2-5; severe neuroforaminal narrowing, moderate stenosis L5-S1	Bilaterally prolonged H reflexes without denervation	Heavy legs, left sided sciatica with walking, standing and sitting	32.8	32.8	0	32.8	32.8	Muscle-energy, McKenzie type extension work	65% improvement	Pt had epidurals and ascribed most of her improvement to them, but PT reported improvement from second of 11 sessions	L

Table 8.3 (continued)

Decision: spondylolisthesis and/or stenosis and HNP

Name	Age	MRI	EMG	Comments	Anatomical	3 min	Difference	Other Side	3 min	Therapy	Outcome	Comments	Side
13	67	Stenosis	Denervation left L5, right L4, bilateral gastrocnemii		40.4	40.4	0	40.5	40.5	Flexion exercises	95%	LBP, bipedal paraesthesias, numbness; left with mild pedal numbness after six sessions	L
14	62	Spondylosisthesis L5-S1, HNP L12	Right L3-4-5, left L5-S1	Chronic sciatica with previous laser surgery L3-4	39.7	40.5	0.8	33.9	NA	Laser surgery L1-2	Initially 60% improvement	Good relief but some pain returned	B
15	64	L4-5 narrowing	Normal	LBP from lifting	32.1	32.1	0	31.2	31.2	McKenzie	50% improvement	Pain returning 2 years later, seeks therapy again	B
16	44	Gr I–II spondylolisthesis	Normal	LBP, buttock pain	29.2	29.2	0	29.3	29.2	Muscloskeletal work	No improvement	Subsequent facet joint: RFA with 85% improvement	B
17	63	Spondylolisthesis, HNP L4-5	Anterior tib	Drop foot	32.7	32.9	0.2	30.1	30.1	McKenzie	98% improvement	Dorsiflexion now 5–/5	R
18	74	Severe stenosis neuroforaminal and narrowing L2-5; severe neuroforaminal narrowing, moderate stenosis L5-S1	Bilateral H reflexes prolonged	Heavy legs	32.8	32.8	0	32.8		Extension/ Epidurals	65% improvement	Lost heavy feeling in legs	L
Mean	61.13				33.64	33.76	0.12	32.81	32.64				
SD	10.09				4.14	4.31	0.28	3.47	3.74				

Table 8.4 Summary of outcome of patients with H reflexes significantly delayed by 3-min extension: those treated for spinal stenosis vs. other conditions (e.g., radiculopathy)

Patients with positionally exacerbated spinal stenosis*		
Improvement (%)	Treated according to 3-min test	Not treated according to the 3-min test
>50	2,3,4,6,8,9 [6]	0
<50	0	5,7 [2]

*Outcome unknown in one case.

Table 8.5 Summary of outcome of patients with H reflexes not significantly delayed by 3-min extension: those treated for radiculopathy vs. other conditions (e.g., spinal stenosis)

Patients without positionally exacerbated spinal stenosis		
Improvement (%)	Treated according to 3 min test (n)	Not treated according to 3-min test (n)
>50	10,11,12,13,14,15,17,18 [8]	0
<50	0	16 [1]

Table 8.6 Patients with and without positionally exacerbated spinal stenosis classified by outcome of treatment according to the results of their 3-min extension test

	All Patients	
Improvement (%)	Treated according to 3-min test	Not treated according to the 3-min test
>50	14	0
<50	0	3

$P < 0.001$

with the extension maneuver. If such a change in the H reflex does occur, one would expect it to shorten, rather than lengthen the latency, yet latency increase is what we have seen in the cases of positionally exacerbated spinal stenosis (PESS). It is possible that a tendency to shorten the latency does work in the opposite direction, obscuring mild increases that might be seen in extension with mild stenosis, and these effects might cancel each other out, but that seems unlikely. There is even evidence that some other muscles that might be activated during extreme extension, such as plantar flexors, homonymous muscles, and those involved in clenching the teeth may moderate the amplitude of the H reflex [8–11]. If that tendency to shorten the H reflex occurred very often, we would expect to see a genuine shortening in normals. In fact, we have seen it only three times in 5 years of testing, and in each of those cases, there was a herniated or bulging disc for which shortening of the H-reflex latency with extension has another, McKenzie-related explanation.

B. Mobility of the peripheral sciatic nerve, cauda equina, and/or lumbosacral plexus might account for some delay. Since the shortest distance between two points is a straight line, the more one's back arches, the further depolarizations along the nerve fibers must travel to reach the conus medullaris. The act of extension might draw the nerve fibers rostrally, requiring the H reflex literally to cover more ground, and therefore yield a greater latency.

   Similarly, drawing out the nerve fibers might reduce saltatory conduction through some effect on the Schwann cells or nodes of Ranvier.

   If either of these factors were telling, one would expect the effect to be proportional to the amount of extension that people were able to muster, not any neuropathology. This did not seem to be the case. Furthermore, this principle would apply nearly equally well to people with and without spinal stenosis. Examination of the MRIs, latency changes, and treatment outcomes does not bear this out.

C. The average age of these probands is quite high. Possibly the neurological specifications of normal function tighten with increasing age, and these patients are not representative of what we would see if we were to administer the 3-min test to younger patients. Stretching the aging rostral spinal cord may affect the more rostral structures' influence on reflex activities below; stretching the rootlets of the cauda equina may affect their conductivity more directly, or some combination of these two elements may add up to the kind of change we see here.

   Again no account of the changes we see here can be based on age, since the entire series is older, those with PESS and those without.

   Furthermore, while the variability of H reflexes does increase with age, no such increase is found in the variability of side-to-side comparisons [1]. The standard deviations used for side-to-side variability have, therefore, application throughout the chronological spectrum.

2. The groups that did not show changes in H-reflex latency with extension are not rigorously analyzed. These patients were examined with the full rigor of clinical diligence but were not selected and randomized for any formal study. They are not age- or description-matched with the stenotic or spondylolisthetic groups. This chapter's work may be looked at as suggestive, as conceptual, but it must be freely admitted that the non-stenotic groups were not analyzed with the detail up to the current canon of scientific investigation. Nevertheless, it is an attempt to make more informed decisions in reasonably common clinical situations in which there really is no proven procedure, and until such studies are conducted, these decisions may be improved by virtue of the methods cited and assessed here and in the next chapter.

   Observing a few applications of the 3-min test might help to develop an intuitive grasp of its possible uses. This group comprises the chapter. The final chapter begins with totally different applications of functional electrodiagnosis that have come up in clinical practice and ends with some advice and guidelines for those who care to use or extend the ideas in this book

References

1. Fritz, JM, Erhard, RE, Delitto, A, Welch, WC, Nowakowski, PE. "Preliminary results of the use of a two-stage treadmill test as a clinical diagnostic tool in the differential diagnosis of lumbar spinal stenosis." *J Spinal Disord.* 1997 Oct;10(5):410–6.
2. Whitman, JM, Flynn, TW, Childs, JD, Wainner, RS, Gill, HE, Ryder, MG, Garber, MB, Bennett, AC, Fritz, JM. "A comparison between two physical therapy treatment programs for patients with lumbar spinal stenosis: a randomized clinical trial." *Spine.* 2007 April 1;32(7):833–4.
3. Whitman, JM, Flynn, TW, Fritz, JM. "Nonsurgical management of patients with lumbar spinal stenosis: a literature review and a case series of three patients managed with physical therapy." *Phys Med Rehabil Clin N Am.* 2003 Feb;14(1):77–101.
4. Fritz, J. "A Nonsurgical Treatment Approach for Patients With Lumbar Spinal Stenosis." *Phys Therapy* 1997 Sep;77(9):964.
5. Sortland, O et al. "Functional myelograpy with metrizamide in the diagnosis of lumbar spinal stenosis." *Acta Radiol.* 1977;355(suppl):42–54.
6. McKenzie, R. *Treat your own Back.* (Paperback) Orthopedic Physical Therapy Product, 1997.
7. Buschbacher, RM. "Normal range for H-reflex recording from the calf muscles." *Am M Phys Med Rehabil.* 1999;78(Suppl):S75–S79.
8. Fisher, MA. AAEM minimonograph #13: "H-reflexes and F waves: physiology and clinical indications." *Muscle Nerve.* 1992;15:1223–33.
9. Tazoe, T, Kida, T, Wasaka, T, Sakamoto, M, Nakajima, T, Nishihira, Y, Komiyama, T. "Attenuation of the effect of remote muscle contraction on the soleus H-reflex during plantar flexion." *Clin Neurophysiol.* 2005 Jun;116(6):1362–9.
10. Nardone, A, Schieppati, M. "Inhibitory effect of the Jendrassik maneuver on the stretch reflex." *Neuroscience.* 2008;156(3):607–17 (Jul 26–Oct 15).
11. Miyahara, T. "Modulation of soleus H-reflex by teeth clenching." *Kokubyo Gakkai Zasshi.* 1991 Dec;58(4):670–86 (Japanese. Read in abstract. PMID: 1795137 MEDLINE).

Chapter 9
Treating Spinal Stenosis Identified by an Evoked Electromyographic Sign: Analysis of the Data

Abstract Because the evocative maneuver of extending the spine for 3 min is used as a decision procedure between therapeutic alternatives, the most persuasive illustration of its efficacy may be case studies. This chapter focuses on the outcome of therapy in dual diagnosis and other cloudy circumstances in which this and other functional maneuvers have helped to select the proper therapeutic approach.

Keywords McKenzie · Cauda Equina · Pronator syndrome · Extreme and prolonged · Claudication · Fusion · Sacral mass

Illustrative Examples

Having looked at the history of electricity in Medicine, and attempted to show the utility of provocative and evocative maneuvers in the physical examination in the first three chapters, and having tried to demonstrate the reasonableness of a more functional approach to nerve conduction studies using such maneuvers in the last five chapters, it is time to cite cases in which a combination of diagnoses present circumstances in which these extensions of the physical examination help determine what will be beneficial to our patients. The 3 min extension test is featured in most of these examples since its main function is to make exactly these distinctions.

The Tale of the Horse's Tail

A 60-year-old actor and proofreader with a history of radical surgery and radiation for prostatic cancer 10 years earlier had been referred directly to PT and had been treated for musculoskeletal lower back pain for 3 weeks when the physical therapist reported sudden onset of bladder incontinence to the physician. When we saw the patient, we noted bilateral plantar sensory deficits. The patient complained that he had been "dragging" his left leg more and more over the past 2 weeks.

L.M. Fishman, A.N. Wilkins, *Functional Electromyography*,
DOI 10.1007/978-1-60761-020-5_9,

We arranged for the therapist to accompany him to a nearby emergency room. It was Friday afternoon; so we gave the therapist our cell-phone numbers. Two hours later we received a call from the ER physician stating that this was cauda equina syndrome, and an emergency MRI would probably be followed by surgery. Two hours later a different emergency room physician called, saying they had given him opiates and were sending him home. Two hours later still the patient was on the phone, telling us his pain was unbearable and that he had collapsed in the hospital parking lot.

We called a nearby pharmacy to arrange oral steroids and sent him to a second hospital's emergency room. We called the MRI facility. The tech, after much coaxing, described a centrally herniated disc at L5-S1 with a fragment "pushing on the cauda equina."

The second emergency room was part of the same hospital network, and so the physician could access the MRI. She said there was too much movement artifact, that the patient was in so much pain he could not hold still that long, but did not believe it was cauda equina. She drained his bladder of 1.6 l of fluid, she told us, and discharged him with an indwelling catheter, firmly convinced that this was overflow incontinence due to some neurological consequence of the prostate surgery 10 years earlier.

We met him at the office early the next day. There was reddish fluid in the leg bag. The steroids, he said, had made the pain 30% better, but the biplantar sensory deficits were still present, and he walked with a poorly compensated Trendelenburg. Furthermore, his glans had reduced sensation, the shaft of the penis had an even greater sensory deficit, but the scrotal sac was hardly affected.

We compared H reflexes in the anatomical position with those in maximal extension. The patient literally gritted his teeth, an identified stimulant of the H reflex [1], and persisted for the full 3 min on each side. The left H reflex was delayed 3.1 ms; the right H reflex was delayed 1.3 ms by the extension maneuver. There was denervation at S1 and quite floridly at S3, but very little at S2. We sent the patient to a neurosurgeon, and spoke with him on the phone about the patient's course and our findings. He agreed about the motion artifact on the first MRI, and waited 3 days for insurance approval for an MRI under anesthesia.

The MRI revealed a large mass in the sacrum, profoundly narrowing it. At biopsy, the cells resembled the prostate cancer of 10 years before. This gave sufficient additional evidence and surgery was performed. Six weeks after the surgery, the patient had only incisional pain and no longer needed Depends.

Stenosis or Thrombosis

A 72-year-old high-functioning lawyer with a long history and recent worsening of right lower back, hip, buttock, and leg pain that intensified with more than 1 block's walking and a cardiac stent, came to us with CT in hand, showing severe stenosis at L3-4, moderate stenosis at L4-5, and significant arthritis narrowing the neuroforamina at those levels as well. He had sensory deficits at both right and left first web-spaces and the dorsal aspects of both feet, with symmetrically reduced patellar and Achilles tendon reflexes. There was no gross weakness. Hand-held Doppler was normal, including provocative arterial and venous tests.

Conventional EMG found a right H reflex of 44.6 and a left of 41.8 ms, positive sharp waves bilaterally at L3-4-5 and S1, and no peripheral signs of denervation. Although the right-sided H reflex was more delayed than the left, there were 2+ positive sharp waves at the right L3-4 and the left L5-S1: we were left in a quandary as to the side on which we should try re-eliciting the H reflex in extension. We changed the electrodes during the 3-min maneuver, and in that way testing both legs took only a few seconds more than 3 min. This was preferable to repeating the maneuver for a total of 6 min.

The right-sided H reflex was prolonged 1.5 ms as the 3-min period came to an end. We took that as a three standard deviation prolongation of the H reflex. The increase followed the exponential-type rise illustrated in Fig. 8.3. We concluded that the patient's complaints were most traceable to stenosis.

The patient was treated with flexion exercises, manual therapy, and abdominal strengthening. He recovered more than 50% within 14 sessions of physical therapy.

Fusion and Confusion

A 39-year-old travel executive and single mother with a diagnosis of Ehlers-Danlos syndrome and lumbar fusion from L3 to S1 five years ago came to us complaining of severe pain located just above the incision site, at L2-3. Range of motion was, of course, restricted in the lumbar spine, but otherwise appeared reasonably normal. Motor strength was 4+/5 in proximal and distal muscles. Apart from left lateral calf and dorsal foot numbness, which had been present for years, there were no sensory abnormalities. The left Achilles tendon reflex was reduced.

CT revealed a reduced disc space at L2-3 and a severely arthritic facet, but in itself that did not distinguish between stenosis, narrowed neuroforamina, and a facet problem. EMG revealed that the left H reflex latency was 2.6 ms longer than the right, the only abnormality apart from paraspinal-positive sharp waves that were no more intense at L2-3 than bilaterally at many lower lumbar levels. These admitted of ambiguous interpretation given the surgical incision. Three minutes' extension further prolonged the left H reflex 1.6 ms. We treated the patient with gentle flexion exercises and skilled manual work that focused on flexion above L3. The patient learned some home exercises and how to engage the paraspinal musculature herself quite quickly. She improved 75%, considerably more than she had in a number of years of therapy.

Evocative Maneuver

A 39-year-old TV and music-recording producer presented after 3 weeks' severe left lower back pain and sciatica that began a few days following a basketball game. There was no prior history of similar complaints. On physical examination, the left

Achilles tendon reflex was mildly reduced, but otherwise his was a normal motor and sensory examination.

After six sessions of physical therapy for paraspinal and hamstring muscle spasm, the patient returned reporting no improvement whatever. His insurance company refused to authorize an MRI. EMG at that time detected positive sharp waves at the L5 paraspinal musculature and a 2.3-ms delay of the left H reflex as compared with the right, though that value did not reach the criterion for absolute abnormality. Still, for side-to-side variation, this was quite significant.

Placing the patient in extension for 3 min *shortened* the H-reflex latency by 0.9 ms. This, along with the EMG findings, suggested neuroforaminal narrowing rather than spinal stenosis or spondylolisthesis, and the patient was treated with McKenzie exercises and other elements in the standard treatment for lateral herniation of the fifth lumbar disc. His pain was reduced 80% within the next 3 weeks. In the meantime, possibly on the strength of the evidence from the EMG, the MRI was authorized and showed an L5 disc herniation on the left.

Aye, Where's the Rub?

A 62-year-old First Amendment lawyer had seen us off and on for several years to alleviate a recurrently nagging back ache. Each time, after a few weeks had passed, and six to eight treatments with them, she was back at the job she never left, but in better condition and without enough pain to motivate continued therapy. That is, until she presented with severe right-sided sciatica and a drop foot that she described as worsening over the past 6 weeks. It took us several minutes to move her into the examining room from where she was silently sitting in the waiting area.

There was 1/5 extension strength in all five toe and right ankle extensors, reduced sensation over the dorsal and posterolateral foot, and a very stiff spine. The physical examination was sharply limited by her pain and immobility, but some essentials did come through: the buttock and sacroiliac joint were non-tender, and there was a steep drop-off in the posterior spinous processes between L4 and L5.

Her pain level and the cloudy timing made EMG inadvisable, but NCV and H reflexes were pursued. A 9 m/s slowing with 20% reduction in compound muscle action potentials was seen in conductions initiated proximal to the right fibular head. Right-sided peroneal H reflex was delayed nearly 3 ms compared to the left, but the posterior tibial H reflexes were symmetrically normal. Placing the patient in 3-min extension (which partially relieved the pain) produced no prolongation of the H reflexes whatever.

We gave her an air-cast, self-tapering steroids and morphine, arranged for an emergency MRI, and offered to drive her to the radiologist. "Don't be ridiculous," she said, and walked out.

Later that morning the faxed MRI report read as follows:

1. "Grade I anterolisthesis of L4 on L5.
2. Critical stenosis at L4-5, with ligamentum flavum hypertrophy and facet arthropathy. Residual canal diameter 4.5 mm.
3. Marked stenosis at L5-S1.
4. Marked bilateral neuroforaminal stenosis with suspected compression upon the exiting right L4 and L5 nerve roots..." We gave her the names of three surgeons and began very cautious physical therapy.

Since the extension relieved her pain in our brief interview, we began her on mild and cautious McKenzie exercises and manual medical therapies in spite of the spondylolisthesis and critical stenosis mentioned so prominently in the MRI report. Whether it were mainly the steroids, the therapy, or a combination of the two, she rapidly became 75–80% better and gained 3−/5 strength in right ankle dorsiflexion in the next 3 weeks. By then she had seen one surgeon who recommended a fusion, and a second that was not sure whether the radiculopathic or stenotic component was mainly responsible for her pain and disability. He cited the fact that her pain was relieved somewhat by extension and its unilateral nature.

Still contemplating surgery, she continued in physical therapy, and we continued the same McKenzie-type treatment and completed the EMG. There was denervation of the right anterior tibialis and peroneus longus but none in the paraspinal musculature. The right peroneal H reflex was still prolonged for more than 3 ms with respect to the left. The peroneal palsy began to look like a major cause of the drop foot, as the lower back pain and proximal sciatic-type pain receded. At 8 weeks she was 95% better, still using the air-cast, with a third surgical opinion that came and went. After 18 months she said "At least for now, any surgical suggestions will be more or less academic."

Recreational Therapy

A 66-year-old retired social worker, a long-time patient, and experienced world traveler who had owned and used a motorcycle for many years, presented with bilateral pseudoclaudication with walking short distances and with sleeping on his stomach. He had given up the motorcycle with our encouragement some time before the pain began. There were no peripheral vascular, sensorimotor, or orthopedic signs. MRI revealed grade-I spondylolisthesis. Standard EMG showed a 1.0 ms delay in the left H reflex, positive sharp waves at left L5, and increased insertional activity in the left gastrocnemius.

Placing the patient in extension for 3 min further prolonged the left H reflex by 1.3 ms. As a consequence, he was given flexion exercises, physical therapy to strengthen core muscles, and Alexander Technique instruction to improve his posture. He left town before we could see him again.

When we did return, he reported that after those 2 weeks of therapy, he was well enough to go to the Far East for several months, but needed to see us again (approximately 1 year later) for further treatment. After those few weeks, he said he was able to walk just about as far as he liked, and reported that he had experienced no sciatica riding a rented motorcycle in the interim.

However, on his return to the United States, he had found that the pain was returning too. He came to us describing pain that developed with walking and became so severe that he took his bicycle even on short errands. When asked, he said that on the bike, there was never any pain.

We speculated that the forward-leaning position that motorcycle riders assume had actually prevented his positionally stenotic spine from giving him problems, while the moderately extended spine of the brisk walker worsened his pain. We explained this to him to highlight the importance of his posture, reiterating what the Alexander therapist had said. That and an abdominal binder has seemed to treat this well ever since.

If It Walks Like a Duck. . .

A large, somewhat overweight 53-year-old news editor presented with severe left-sided lower back pain and sciatica. The pain was worse with sitting, which is what he was obliged to do most workdays.

On physical examination, there was weakness in toe walking on the left, with a sensory deficit on the lateral and posterolateral left foot and heel, and along the distal lateral thigh. The left Achilles tendon reflex was present, but only half the strength that was found at the right. Straight leg raises were positive on the right and left at 60° and 45°, respectively.

The MRI showed not only significant spinal stenosis, but also a central disc herniation at L4-5, and a left paracentral disc at L5-S1.

Conventional EMG showed a 4.1 ms delay in left posterior tibial H-reflex latency, without evidence of frank paraspinal or peripheral denervation. The question was whether this man's condition were due to the foraminal effects of the L5 disc herniation or due to the central stenoses brought on by the central herniations and the spinal stenosis described on the MRI, or due to some combination of both.

Placing the patient in 3-min extension *shortened* the H reflex quite quickly (after 90 s) by 1.6 ms, strongly suggesting that the herniated disc at L5-S1 was responsible for at least the larger portion of his pain.

He was treated with McKenzie exercises, and he found himself more than 50% improved within a few weeks.

Discussion: One might have suspected that the L5-S1 disc were responsible for most of the patient's pain after noting the reduced left Achilles tendon reflex and the sensory changes restricted to the left side, but there was certainly room for doubt, especially since both a central and a paracentral herniation were present. The 3-min test gave added confidence to a treatment that would have been exactly wrong if the stenosis had turned out to be the dominant pain generator. The fact that extension actually shortened the H-reflex latency strengthened the case for the herniated disc, but even the absence of any prolongation would have tended to promote McKenzie exercises here rather that flexion.

Small Change

A 61-year-old five-feet tall 170-pound music teacher's aide with a history of moderately severe spastic cerebral palsy and childhood right trimalleolar fusion had suffered progressively severe gait disorder over the past 10 years, leading to falls that generally occurred as she was ascending higher curbs after crossing the street. There was little lower extremity spasticity, but hip flexion was moderately limited after one such fall resulted in a left acetabular fracture. Her gait had begun to deteriorate more quickly over the past 6 months, and close examination revealed that the left plantar- and dorsiflexors, critical for mounting and descending curbs in her situation, had begun to weaken.

MRI showed a fair-sized central and left paracentral disc herniation at L4-5. EMG showed bilateral denervation of the anterior tibialis, gastrocnemius, and peroneus longus, more severe on the left than the right. Normal rehabilitation techniques had been employed many times with this intelligent and thoughtful woman, and had increased her ranges of motion and reduced her discomfort on numerous occasions. This time they were nearly useless.

We considered surgery, but the question was, for what? Was spinal stenosis or neuroforaminal narrowing responsible for her new problem? Since her spinal range of motion was indeed critical for safe ambulation, and getting up from the low stools the children sat on in her school was an absolute prerequisite for her job, a fusion procedure with its long immobilization was particularly undesirable. Time in the hospital was not going to help her mobility, strength, or job-situation either.

We had seen her at various times and for various problems over more than a decade, and there were two previous electrophysiological examinations in which extension had produced insignificant delay in her H reflexes. A new study, done just before she entered PT for a herniated disc, showed a delay of 0.4 ms. She continued to deteriorate. Two months and three near-falls later, we performed the 3-min test again, this time showing a larger delay (2.1 ms). A subsequent MRI showed the development of significant spinal stenosis at the level of the disc.

We reversed our treatment, now using flexion exercises, manual therapy, and gait training emphasizing mild flexion. She improved 60% within a short time, did not enter the hospital, but rather went back to work at the school.

Discussion: This is a case of rapidly developing spinal stenosis, which rose from slight to severe in the course of a few months. Extension therapy had possibly been worse than useless, and seemed to be exacerbating her condition. The serially increasing H-reflex latencies with extension were indications that spinal stenosis was behind her mounting pain and disability, and gave sufficient cause for a confirmatory MRI.

We will now present some cases of greater complexity in which the 3-min test and the FAIR test may both come into play, and where the *absence* of positive results to these tests is helpful in ruling out potential diagnoses, helping to guide treatment.

When Therapy Is Not Enough

A high-functioning 80-year-old retired behavioral psychologist presented with bilateral sciatica that worsened with walking. His wife was functioning as a gait-aid as well as a companion.

The patient had not improved in 1 month of McKenzie type physical therapy at another facility. At that point an MRI was performed, showing significant stenosis at L3-4, and herniated discs there at L4-5 and at L5-S1. The patient had transforaminal injections at L4-L5 and L5-S1, which gave him some relief. After 2 months the benefits began to wane, and he considered acupuncture, yoga, and, he said, if these failed, then surgery.

The question of what surgery would be appropriate was what brought the patient to us. Early in the history and physical examination it became clear that extension, even straightening up, intensified the pain. EMG revealed no H-reflex delay but bilateral denervation potentials at the paraspinal muscles of L4-5 and L5-S1, and most of all at the left L3-L4. The 3-min extension test was very difficult, because extension was quite painful for the patient. However, it was not necessary to hold the very slight extension that the patient could manage—less than 20°—there was 2.6 ms and 3.7 ms delay in the left and right posterior tibial H reflexes after 10 and 30 s, respectively.

This dramatically highlighted the contribution that spinal stenosis was making to his bilateral sciatica. The fact that the major denervation was at L3-4, but the pain was sciatic in nature pointed to the same conclusion. He sought surgical consultation.

Less Was Probably More

An 87-year-old totally lucid woman with 76° thoracolumbar rotatory levoscoliosis had severe left-sided lower back pain with standing. The apex of the curve was L2. When she sat down or lay down, the pain vanished. Although there certainly was a notable rotatory component and a significant postural deformation, no respiratory symptoms had occurred.

She had been in physical therapy to improve her ambulation and balance, but it had done little to relieve her pain over 3 months of treatment. She had been convinced to see an orthopedic surgeon regarding the scoliosis, but one important factor was whether spinal stenosis were present. MRI revealed a mild to moderately narrowed intraspinal space, but the question was whether the scoliosis had exacerbated the compressive forces of the bony spine on the cauda equina.

She was unable to stay in the extended position at first, but after one try and a rest, she did a yeoman's job, and we found no prolongation of the otherwise normal and symmetrical H reflexes in 3-min extension.

We sent word to the scoliosis surgeon that there was no electrophysiological evidence of stenosis; a Cottrell-Dubosset type procedure was performed without any work on the inner canal, and a fusion was not done. The patient is now

70% improved with respect to the scoliosis and has very little left-sided pain with standing.

A Long Shot

A 42-year-old real estate broker came to us with back pain radiating to his right lower extremity. The pain was much worse standing, and nearly vanished when he sat down. MRI showed a broad-based disc bulge at L4-5 with minimal anterolisthesis at that level, and a bilateral pars defect. There was mild central spinal stenosis and severe bilateral foraminal narrowing due to the asymmetrically lateralizing disc material that was significantly exaggerated on the right, combined with facet and ligamentum flavum hyptertrophy. In addition there was a superiorly extruded disc fragment that appeared to contact and displace the descending right L4 nerve root. Over the next month, instead of improving with physical therapy, the lower back pain worsened. In August he lifted a heavy object and heard a "pop." Thereafter there were stabbing pains, paraesthesias, and numbness in his right lateral shin when he stood up or walked, but just about absent when he was lying down or seated.

The patient then had two transforaminals, the first of which reduced his pain from 9/10 to 5/10, but the sensory deficit continued unchanged. EMG revealed bilateral denervation at L4-5-S1, and the right anterior tibialis. The patient had a microdiscectomy 6 weeks later, then a second course of three transforaminal steroid injections, and then a second microdiscectomy.

When he returned to us 60 days later, he reported that apart from the first epidural, none of this had helped him very much. He was in 7–8/10 pain when he was standing or walking, still with the sciatica, the sensory changes, and only minimally able to work. In fact there was now sensory loss in the anterior thigh, and his condition became unbearable after walking less than one block or standing for more than 25–30 min. He sought advice on whether to undergo a third surgery that would fuse L4-5.

EMG again turned up denervation in the right anterior tibialis that was no more intense than it had been 6 months before, with progression neither to the vastus medialis nor to the L3-4 paraspinal musculature. The right and left H reflexes were symmetrically normal. We kept the electrodes in place on the soleus at the right medial calf, turned on our timer, and asked the patient to stand, evoking H reflexes every 30 s. The pain was quite severe by 22 min, when we stopped. The H reflex actually shortened by 2.4 ms during that time period, showing the characteristically accelerating late change in latency that we had seen in many other cases, but in the opposite direction.

We reasoned that if the spondylolisthesis had worsened, then the latency would have increased as the L5-S1 fibers that crossed the centrally bulging disc at L4 became compressed. Rather, the centrally bulging disc seemed to have been retracted by 22 min standing, actually making for the reduction in H-reflex latency. There was no neuropathological need for a fusion, the problem was still at L4-5, and not necessarily related any more to the herniation. There had been no extension of the neurological damage. We sent the patient to an anesthesiologist to evaluate him for a transforaminal injection. The anesthesiologist reviewed the imaging studies and the unchanged EMG and had another idea. Radiofrequency ablation of the medial branch at L4 reduced the pain 85–90%.

Embarrassment of Riches

A 53-year-old child psychologist had 8/10 to 9/10 left-more-than-right sciatica for nearly 10 months. She had seen us for the last three of those months; we had been treating her for piriformis syndrome, given a positive FAIR test, and a negative MRI 1 month after the pain began. We had not helped her much; she consented to a second MRI.

We were surprised, and in a way relieved to see that the second MRI showed disc disease at L4-5 and L5-S1 causing bilateral foraminal narrowing, especially at L4-5 and particularly on the left. There was also moderate spinal stenosis at both levels. Ironically, we were quite glad because it appeared that there was something that we had missed. . .something new to treat that might help her.

Unfortunately, the new information left us with an embarrassment of riches: there were three conditions, and not at all with the same treatment: extension (which the therapist had tried) would relieve the discal disease that narrowed the neuroforamina but worsen spinal stenosis; flexion might be valuable for the stenotic component but might extend the disc pathology; and the type of twisting that we have found so successful for piriformis syndrome might worsen the discs' condition and could not be trusted with stenosis either.

We repeated the EMG. In the anatomical position the left posterior tibial H reflex was prolonged just under three standard deviations beyond the mean at 1.20 ms; peroneal conductions had low amplitudes, particularly on the left, but otherwise nerve conduction velocities and action potentials were within normal limits. EMG turned up 2+ positive sharp waves and 1+ fibrillation potentials at the left L4-5 but not elsewhere in bilateral studies. At least there appeared to be a neuroforaminal pain generator involving the posterior more than the anterior primary division at the left L4. But what about the stenosis and piriformis syndrome?

We compared the posterior tibial and peroneal H-reflexes' latencies in the anatomical position with the same reflexes in flexion, adduction, and internal rotation (FAIR test). The posterior tibial H reflex was replicably prolonged 2.6 ms, and the wave became bifid, the second, larger component peaking another 2.2 ms later. The peroneal H reflex vanished altogether with the FAIR maneuver. We then measured the left posterior tibial H reflex in the prone position and every 30 s thereafter with the patient in fairly extreme extension (see Fig. 8.1).

After 1.5 min, the reflex was delayed 1.1 ms, and remained so for the rest of the test (another 1.5 min). We had to find a way to quantify these three separate abnormalities and it was as follows

1. *The positive sharp waves and fibrillation potentials at the left L4-5.* We have never seen a study estimating the probability of this happening "by chance," but the denervation potentials were fairly impressive. Also there was the almost significant prolongation of the left H reflex at rest. Together these implicated the pathological disc at L4-5 as stenosing the neuroforamen and compressing the L5 root.
2. The 2.6-ms prolongation of the H reflex by the FAIR position was more than four standard deviations beyond the mean, suggesting a severe piriformis syndrome.
3. The 1.1-ms delay of the H reflex by 3-min extension was just more than two standard deviations beyond the mean for side-to-side variation in normals, consistent with mild/moderate spinal stenosis.

Reviewing the whole situation, including the standard deviations beyond the mean of each metric, we concluded that the positive sharp waves and the prolongation of the left posterior tibial H reflex in flexion, adduction, and internal rotation were the most significant abnormalities, indicating the likely major pathogenetic mechanisms at work producing in the patient's pain. We resolved to intensify our treatment of the piriformis syndrome. We gave her a trigger point injection into the piriformis muscle under EMG guidance. However, we had seen other pathology too, arranged for her to have epidurals at L4-5, and split our work in PT between the piriformis muscle and gentle, careful extension techniques according to the methods of McKenzie. Within a few days her pain was 1/10, and she held off on the epidurals.

Less There Than Met the MRI

A 67-year-old partially retired gold and antiques dealer came to our office with lower back pain, loss of left more than right anterior thigh sensation, and a recent MRI showing moderate to severe spinal stenosis at L2-3. He had already had a full EMG when the pain troubled him some years ago, and another one just a month ago at another facility, both showing a sensorimotor axonal and demyelinating polyneuropathy, and denervation only of the left anterior tibialis. He had undergone two epidural injections and physical therapy for the stenosis, but nothing seemed to help.

On physical examination there was a very mild, almost subtle reduction of sensory acuity at the dorsal right foot, with positive left straight leg raise at 70°, versus 80° on the right. These were the only positive findings, apart from reduced movement of the sacroiliac joints on flexion. We decided to repeat the H reflexes, comparing the latencies after 3-min extension with what we first found in the anatomical position. EMG had been done repeatedly, but we felt the 3-min extension test might yield something useful to him. There was a significant delay in left H reflex versus the right in the anatomical position, but no further delay in right or left posterior tibial or peroneal H reflexes in 3 min of extension. We then felt it necessary to go further electrodiagnostically. EMG revealed nearly florid denervation of the paraspinal muscles at left L3-4 and significant right-sided denervation at the same level. We sent him to physical therapy for McKenzie technique exercises. Within 6 weeks he was 95% better.

Now You See It, Now You Don't, Oh, There It Is Again

A 37-year-old lawyer left his forearm crutches at the door to our office. He had just come to New York, where he planned to work for 8 weeks, and found he suddenly could not walk more than 10 feet without experiencing 9/10 pain in the left side of his lower back, his left buttock, and the leg.

There was weakened dorsiflexion, sensory loss at the first web space and at the dorsal, lateral and posterior foot, and distal lateral calf, with paraesthesias in roughly the same distribution. His left piriformis muscle was nearly exquisitely tender and impressively tight.

He was in so much pain, and it was so soon after onset that we restricted our electrodiagnostic examination to left-sided H reflexes. There was a delay of 2.6 ms when the patient was placed in flexion, adduction, and internal rotation (FAIR test).

We injected the motor point of the piriformis muscle with steroid and Marcaine, and began PT for piriformis syndrome. We also sent him for an MRI because of the severity of his pain.

The next week he returned without the crutches, but still far from totally better. Now he could walk a block or two. We further encouraged him to get the MRI. When it came back a few days later, it revealed a large left-sided L5-S1 disc.

A full EMG again showed a 2.6 ms delay in FAIR test, but a whopping 6.10 ms delay of left versus right H reflexes in the anatomical position. We found denervation of the L5-S1 paraspinal muscles as well as the gastrocnemius, anterior tibialis, and peroneus longus, all confined to the left side.

We concluded that the major source of the patient's problem came from the disc, sent him for two transforaminal injections, and he was 60% better by the time we saw him 2 weeks later. He was scheduled for the third transforaminal the next day, and booked to return to the Midwest a few days later. At that point, he had sensory deficits at the left lateral dorsal and posterolateral foot and distal lateral calf. There was some buttock tenderness.

He wanted to know whether he should consider surgery, continue physical therapy, or what. We repeated the H reflexes, finding both the posterior tibial and peroneal symmetrically normal. The 6.10 ms delay on the left was utterly gone. On the contrary, the left posterior tribial and peroneal H reflexes were now 3.1 and 5.8 ms delayed by flexion, adduction, and internal rotation. The piriformis syndrome appeared to be back.

Being a functional diagnosis, piriformis syndrome can disappear and then reappear very much like a headache. Unlike a headache, it is more than a symptom: it has distinct pathogenetic characteristics and can be diagnosed and treated successfully.

We wrote him a prescription for physical therapy consistent with that diagnosis. We have not heard from him since, apart from learning that he had the third transforaminal injection the next day. Given the studies in Chapter 7, he has an 80% chance of being at least 50% better.

Ex Pluribus Unum

Simple Solutions When There Were Too Many Diagnoses

A 53-year-old public accountant presented with left-sided sciatica and pain at the sole of the foot and distal lateral calf that appeared with straight leg raise. She had seen us some years before, when we diagnosed piriformis syndrome and had succeeded in helping her with treatment for that condition. She had had a normal MRI 1 year ago, when the current complaint surfaced.

The physical examination did show mild sensory deficit at the left lateral plantar surface and up the posterolateral calf almost to the knee.

Apart from sural sensory nerve action potentials that were 40% lower on the left than the right, conventional EMG was normal, as was the piriformis test, and 3 min of extension. Because of this, we carried the EMG into the sacral musculature, where nearly florid denervation was seen at S2-3 and in the left peroneus longus.

We concluded that this was a sacral radiculopathy and attributed the sural sensory nerve action potential to an aftermath of the piriformis syndrome. The peroneal denervation could be due to either cause. McKenzie-type exercises helped the patient 80% within 6 weeks.

Asymmetrical on Both Sides

A 45-year-old artistic director presented with bilateral sciatica and intermittent lower back pain, the latter for 20 years. The MRI showed grade I retrolisthesis at L5-S1 and mild/moderate stenosis at L4-5.

Standard EMG was totally normal; 3 min of extension did not change H reflexes at all, but placing the patient in flexion, adduction, and internal rotation delayed the otherwise normal right posterior tibial H reflex by 3.9 ms. The left H reflex was also prolonged by the FAIR maneuver, but less so.

We treated the patient for piriformis syndrome bilaterally and she improved 90% within a few weeks.

A Long-Standing Problem with Sitting

A 41-year-old writer's left-sided sciatica was not improving after seeing several physical therapists, a yoga therapist, having extensive acupuncture, and 15 treatments with us. We had begun with McKenzie technique and had employed muscle–energy and strain/counterstrain techniques and several other methods. He was beginning to have trouble concentrating with pain he ranked as 6–7/10 and emphasized that it was decidedly worse with sitting. The MRI showed retrolisthesis at L1-2 and L2-3, which was not consistent with a previous EMG that reported mild denervation in bilateral L4-5 paraspinal musculature.

We repeated just the H reflexes in prone position and after 3-min extension. The left posterior tibial H reflex was delayed 1.0 ms after that time in repeated trials. The other posterior tibial and neither peroneal H reflexes were prolonged at all. Reasoning that the spondylolisthesis at higher levels must be compressing the rootlets in the cauda equina that were associated with L4-5-S1 rather than L1-2-3 dermatomes, we concluded that spinal stenosis was a significant pain generator, and treated him with flexion exercises and abdominal strengthening work.

He improved 80% within 2 weeks, and given a flexion routine and an abdominal binder, he has been able to sit at his desk and write from that time to this.

Less There Than Meets the MRI

A working 83-year-old walked slowly into the office with a bilaterally circumductive gait, and told us her legs felt increasingly heavy over the past few months. She also complained of paraesthesias and posterior calf pain that developed after walking 5–10 min. The neurological examination was essentially normal, apart from the gait, with 4/5 strength in all four extremities, no sensory changes, and normal reflexes.

The patient was denied an MRI at first, but X rays of the lumbar and cervical spine revealed extensive osteophytic narrowing of neuroforamina, especially at L1-2-3 and anterior subluxation of C4 on C5 and C7 on T1. EMG revealed delay of the H reflexes in the anatomical position but suggested no further narrowing with 3-min extension.

We began her on a non-specific program of Alexander technique, modalities, and pelvic stabilization with work on the sacroiliac joint at first, since there was no real hint on where to focus physical therapy apart from the arthritis and spondylolistheses. After 4 weeks and perhaps 30% improvement, the MRI was approved. There were disc protrusions at every level from L1-S1 with severe bilateral neuroforaminal narrowing and moderate to severe central canal stenosis at every single level, and mild rotatory lumbar levoscoliosis to boot.

We repeated the 3-min test, this time encouraging a maximal extension effort on the part of this cooperative patient with severe arthritis. She did her best, and the test was still flatly negative.

We treated her with McKenzie exercises for simple neuroforaminal encroachment, and with that and the Alexander Technique she became 60–70% improved within four sessions.

The Woman with Everything

A tall and amply padded 65-year-old woman came with left buttock pain and mild sciatica, with a MRI from her private physician in hand. It showed spondylolisthesis superimposed on a congenitally narrow canal, with some ligamentum flavum and facet hypertrophy as well as bilateral neuroforaminal narrowing at L4-5 and L5-S1, with markedly arthritic facet joints at the latter level.

EMG showed denervation at the left L5 paraspinal musculature and a mildly delayed left H reflex that was further delayed 2.8 ms in 3 min of extension.

We treated her with flexion exercises, manual therapy, and some postural work and she became 85% better within 3 months. At that point we repeated the 3-min test and found a 1.5 ms delay of H reflexes after 3 min of maximal extension.

He Who Hesitates Was Right

A 53-year-old working at a non-profit called the office at 4:30 on Friday, describing unbearable pain and requesting an emergency appointment. We stayed a little late, and when he arrived, there was no question about the terrible pain. Here was a 6-foot 6-inch well-muscled man it was uncomfortable just to look at. The pain needed no further documentation; the question was what caused it. There was numbness of the left lateral foot and lateral calf. These sensory changes were new, though the pain had been developing over a few days following a scrub basketball game with substantially younger participants.

It was too soon for EMG to detect the extent of this injury, but we did bilateral H reflexes, finding a large delay on the affected left side in both the posterior tibial and peroneal branches of the sciatic nerve.

Given the speed at which the pain and sensory deficits had developed, we recommended an emergency MRI. The insurance company refused, and the patient told us he could not afford the cost of the procedure himself.

We gave him oral steroids, Percocet, and our cell-phone number. He did not call, but showed up for physical therapy on Monday, really no better, but at least no worse. The insurance company approved the MRI within a week: it revealed a large left-sided herniated disc at L4-5 causing left-sided neuroforaminal compression and moderate central stenosis. We began physical therapy of the McKenzie type and gave him the telephone numbers of three people who do epidurals and of three neurosurgeons.

Three weeks later, after PT and the first epidural, his pain was 30–40% better. His appointments with the surgeons were coming up, and he stayed in PT.

Three weeks and another epidural later, his left-sided sciatica and sensory deficit were gone, but two new events had taken their place: his right leg was now bothering him quite a bit, and two of the three surgeons had recommended a fusion to treat the spinal stenosis.

At that point we repeated the H reflexes and the EMG, comparing the H reflexes at rest. This yielded a significant 2.5 ms prolongation of the left tibial H reflex in the prone position, with no change after almost 4 min of quite extreme extension. There was no further delay. EMG showed paraspinal denervation at the right L4-5-S1 and the left L5-S1, without appendicular involvement. We kept him in physical therapy, stressing McKenzie-type exercises in spite of the spinal stenosis seen on the MRI, and suggested another, this time transforaminal injection.

Within another 2 weeks he was 85% better in his own estimation, and had cancelled his third surgical appointment in time for it to be filled by someone who needed it more than he.

Reference

1. Miyahara, T "*Modulation of soleus H-reflex by teeth clenching*". *Kokubyo Gakkai Zasshi*. 1991 Dec;58(4):670–86 (Japanese. Read in abstract. PMID: 1795137 MEDLINE).

Chapter 10
Extending Dynamic Electrodiagnosis: Application to Common and Uncommon Conditions

Abstract Having sketched the historical and logical context for electrodiagnosis and diagnoses of exclusion. we have applied electrodiagnostic techniques to elucidate two of those elusive near-diagnostic entities, and to distinguish between the clinical import of two others with similar symptoms and contrary treatments. We now turn to diagnoses that are beyond even diagnoses of exclusion: idiosyncratic or even unique clinical situations in which the same approach has been helpful. We begin by sketching out some guidelines, and end with an exhortation for others to try out these techniques, but harboring the suspicion that other electromyographers have solved problems in similar ways, and constructed other equally valid principles of their own.

Keywords Scapula · Pectoralis major and minor · Auxillary muscles of respiration

Other Uses of Functional Electromyography

Individuals who see value in using provocative and evocative maneuvers in making the diagnosis of thoracic outlet syndrome, piriformis entrapment, and spinal stenosis, and perhaps even some people who do not, may appreciate wider application of the principles that guided those studies. In the final chapter we steer the focus to unstudied and unmuddied waters. Functional methods may help detect other positionally sensitive conditions, incipient carpal tunnel syndrome, early ulnar entrapment at the medial epicondyle or by the lateral head of the flexor carpi ulnaris or the tunnel of Guyon, and other entrapments before they become disabling. This may help people employed in sedentary and high-action jobs to detect repetitive stress due to postural or dysergonomic situations early enough to prevent a good deal of pain, and possibly surgery. Performance-oriented people, and anyone engaged in frequently repetitive tasks may be able to recognize mild injuries and stave off more serious ones through these methods.

Provocative and evocative electrophysiological techniques may also bring out early suprascapular nerve palsy, early peroneal palsy, pronator syndrome, and pressure at the arcade of Frohse before they hamper performance. They are particularly

L.M. Fishman, A.N. Wilkins, *Functional Electromyography*,

DOI 10.1007/978-1-60761-020-5_10,

common in musicians, athletes, and dancers. In all cases, attention to the patient's technique, be it in word processing or throwing a slider, and posture, whether in working a video-editing device, starting a *pas-de-deux* or snatching a rebound, may identify the cause and stimulate practicing a change in behavior before there is a disabling injury, and practice itself becomes impossible.

Some of these cases are common enough to be studied under conditions similar to what we described in Chapters 4, 6, and 8. But some are rare and must be dealt with on the *ad hoc* basis that we began to present here in the closing pages of Chapter 9. We have not had an opportunity to view any of them in a systematic way; we present more them here in the manner we encountered them, intending the material in this chapter to guide the electromyographer who comes up against previously unstudied clinical situations in which these methods might be helpful. In some of these medical vignettes the interplay of electrodiagnosis and the different aspects of clinical medicine will be evident: electrodiagnosis, like the physical examination it extends, is a dynamic part of the total effort to diagnose and heal the patient.

Resources

In the physical examination, physicians have the opportunity to compare pain or function in the anatomical or non-stressed position with what provocative maneuvers bring about. In straight-leg-raise position, it is perfectly unacceptable for the patient to reply "My back still hurts." The question is whether something new happens. The strategy is always to compare some variable's value in the anatomical position with what happens in the provocative maneuver—is it, the maneuver, responsible for anything new? In the physical examination, when performing the straight leg raise, one looks for the location and intensity of pain. But in electromyography, the question is further refined: how much do things have to change to be significant when there are no studies and there are no standards?

We recommend the following three types of measure, depending upon what is available.

1. For H reflexes, F waves and motor and sensory conductions, there is often a *range of standard deviations* or *97th percentile values of side-to-side variation* that can be used. If the provocative maneuver has no actual impact, then one right-sided value of an electrophysiological measure and another right-sided value of that same measure ought to come out as close or closer together than a comparison of right with left. As we have said too often already, two values on one side should not be any further apart than that! At least two and preferably three standard deviations beyond the mean or the equivalent would securely delimit an abnormal value.
2. In cases where such norms are not available, or not applicable, then *testing the unaffected side and comparing the variation brought out by the provocative maneuver there* with what was seen on the affected side may present a

meaningful way to estimate just how unusual the discrepancy in the affected side's values are. Consulting tables of *related* side-to-side standard deviations is useful in gauging significance in a general way too.

3. But these two situations do not exhaust the possibilities. There are bilateral cases without norms, and cases of amputees, and extremities, contralateral and ipsilateral, that are injured in different but relevant ways that make the two extremities incomparable. In this type of case, one wants to get some idea of what is significant. For example, in seeking incipient carpal tunnel syndrome in an upper extremity amputee, where overuse is not unlikely, one starts with what is known: the lowest abnormal distal latency is usually labeled at 4.0–4.5 ms. Normal distal motor latencies are usually set around 3.5 ms. The difference is approximately 1 ms. Now if a provocative maneuver such as flexion at the wrist raises median distal motor latency from 2.5 to 3.9—1.4 ms—one might suspect that it is significant.

In these circumstances, separating out the dependent and independent variables, and *systematically varying the independent variable while seeking progressive changes in the dependent variable*, gives one an electrophysiologically meaningful indication of pathology. For example, an engineer with a right Erb's palsy acquired 20 years before, began having difficulties raising his left index finger during a computer-aided design project. There were fleeting paraesthesias at the first web space, but no weakness on the clinical examination.

We did respective radial motor-posterior interosseous and sensory conductions from the posterolateral upper arm and the lateral cubital fossa. They were normal at rest, and corresponded almost exactly with the NCV (but not the CMAPs) we found on the right. Comparing the left-sided radial motor nerve conduction velocities and CMAPs at rest with the values obtained with moderate and with extreme-and-prolonged elbow flexion and wrist extension (shoulder flexed to 45° and forearm horizontal) showed an inverse relationship between these conditions and NCV with progressively declining CMAPs. MRI showed significant stricture neither at the arcade of Frohse nor elsewhere. We thought that progressive entrapment might occur over time as the radial nerve emerges from the spiral groove and is tethered as it pierces the intermuscular septum. We used myofascial and manual medical techniques with modalities. Along with changes in the patient's seating arrangement and lowering his computer's wrist-pad, we alleviated the problem (Figs. 10.1, 10.2, and 10.3).

Memoirs of a Snapping Scapula

In the seventh grade, this healthy captain of the swim team complained that her right scapula went "click" in free-style competition. Imaging and clinical tests were normal, and we advised her to build up her subscapularis (bilaterally) to cushion the scapula in its rapid and powerful movements against the posterior ribs.

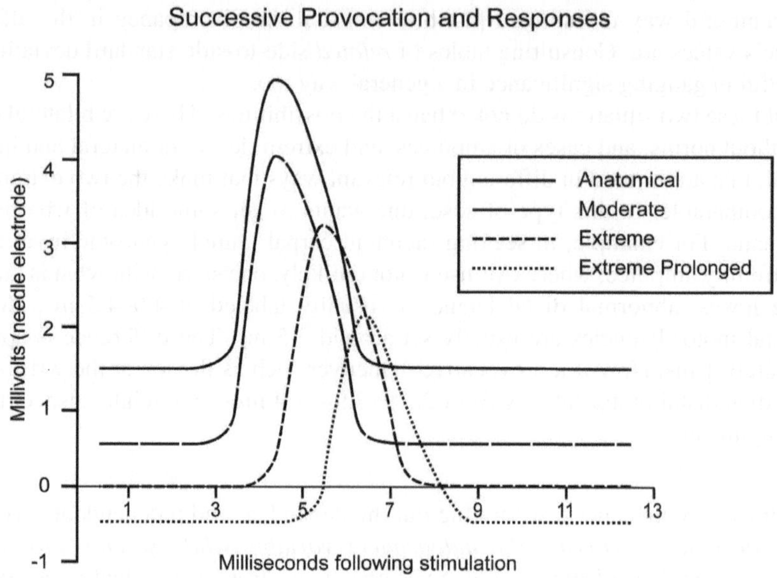

Fig. 10.1 Graph of DML of conductions from the cubital fossa and the spiral groove to extensor indicis proprius in the anatomical position, in moderate, and in prolonged, in extreme, and in prolonged extreme elbow flexion and wrist extension. With successively more extreme provocation the response to stimulation proximal to the septal piercing became successively more delayed and smaller

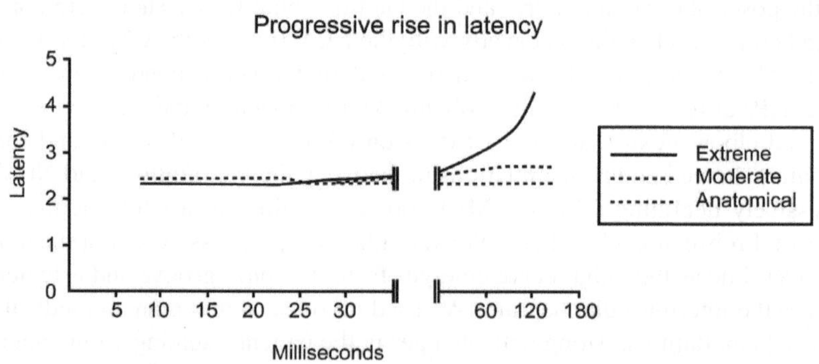

Fig. 10.2 The exponential rise in proximal or distal latency may appear only after increased stress, which must always be restrained by considerations of safety and patient tolerance

Contrary to what we advised, she had a small surgery that tightened the levator scapula and some other muscles of the shoulder girdle, and successfully eliminated the snap.

Ten years later, she came to us again, 3 weeks before her marriage. Again, abducting the right shoulder was the problem. This time abduction caused posterior thoracic clicking and also pain.

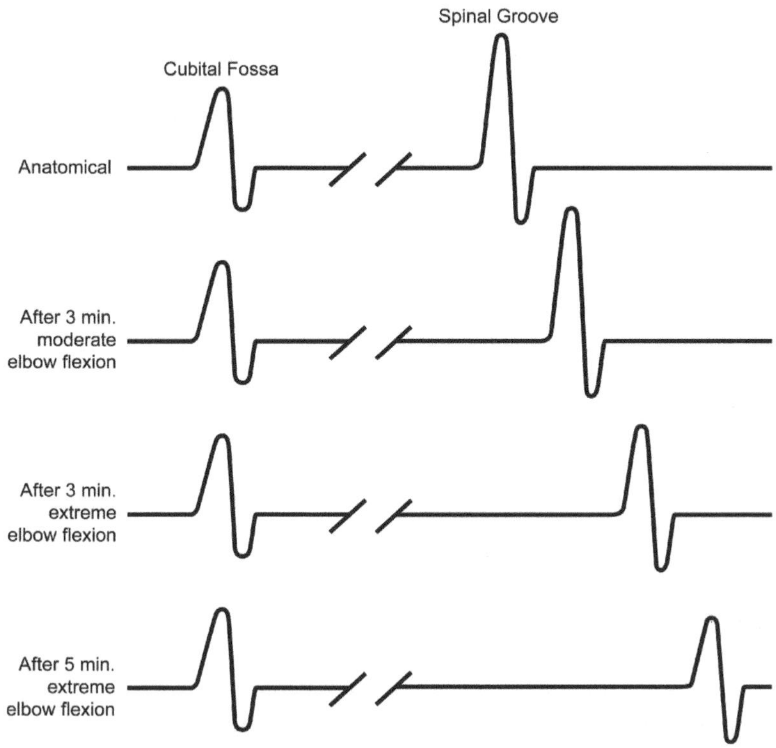

Fig. 10.3 Extreme and prolonged elbow flexion and wrist extension mirrored the circumstances under which the pathology occurred. This may not be the strongest type of evidence, but it may be the strongest possible in the clinical circumstance. Still the co-varying of independent and dependent variables supports the essential validity of any provocative test

MRI of the region suggested that there had been surgery, but that the shoulder and brachial plexus were normal. There was no evidence of unusual structure, osteochondroma, or rotator cuff tear. But of course the problem was with *moving* the shoulder.

The patient calmly abducted the arm up to 75°, then winced with a click and a pain she located at the upper lateral scapular region. The painful clicking was reproduced by movement of the humerus in flexion, provided the scapula moved as well. Extension did not reproduce these phenomena. When we put mild pressure on the teres minor, the clicking stopped completely in spite of movement of both bones.

EMG first definitively identified the muscle as the external rotator the teres minor, and conduction studies along the axillary nerve originating at Erb's point showed a prolongation of 1.1 ms with reasonably extreme external rotation. This did not happen with conductions to the deltoid.

EMG showed polyphasia in the teres minor but not in the deltoid, nor elsewhere.

We tried tightening the pectoralis major through bracing both arms tightly on a table, so that on maximal inhalation the pectoralis minor would act as an auxiliary muscle of respiration and lift the ribs, possibly causing entrapment between the clavicle and the first rib. There was no increase in proximal motor latencies to either the deltoid or the teres minor.

We concluded that the difficulty was entrapment of the branch of the axillary nerve that serves the teres minor and was due to that muscle lifting the scapula rather than simply externally rotating the humerus. It was too weak compared to the muscles such as the deltoid and pectorals that moved the arm in contrary directions and weaker than the internal rotators such as the biceps and even the teres major. Therefore, it was dragged along with them rather than stabilizing the humerus in flexion

We set about a program to strengthen the teres minor through resisted external rotation with the upper arm in 90° abduction, the elbow bent 90°, and the forearm horizontal. We also encouraged the patient specifically to engage the muscle, intending to increase her control over its errant contractions. By the wedding day, the clicking and the pain were subdued 40–50%.

Triple Trouble

A 48-year-old publishing manager was referred by an internist as a "please fit in" emergency. About 10 days previously he had felt a little right lower back pain that developed into 9/10 pain with sciatica within a few days, and brought him to the emergency ward of a nearby hospital 12 h before appearing at our door. In the emergency ward, they seemed to think it was psoriatic arthritis and gave him hydrocodone. He called us terror-stricken outside the hospital in unbearable pain less than an hour later.

There was a history of psoriasis, but no other relevant conditions.

He bravely waited half an hour in our front office, then hobbled in, using a straight cane more in case he started to fall than as an actual aid to ambulation.

There was severe buttock pain with only moderate tenderness, and while heel walking was normal, toe walking on the right foot was impossible. There was numbness of the lateral dorsal foot and distal lateral calf and an absent right patellar and Achilles tendon reflex.

While it was only 10 days from the first symptom, EMG seemed mandatory to sort this out. There were dramatically prolonged right posterior tibial and peroneal H reflexes in the anatomical position, and an even more dramatic prolongation (3.9 ms) in the FAIR position.

The EMG 10 days out showed fibrillation potentials at L5 bilaterally and positive sharp waves in the right medial gastrocnemius.

There was evidence here of both piriformis syndrome and radiculopathy, and the radiculopathic evidence might not have been fully visible at this juncture. The patient's pain had subsided to 4–5/10 while he laid in left lateral decubitus during the testing, which mitigated against piriformis syndrome being the most significant condition on clinical grounds.

In order to estimate the relative contributions of each condition, we used the degree of flexion, adduction, and internal rotation as independent variable and stretched the piriformis muscle progressively as we educed H reflexes.

We found a regular and progressive delay in the H reflexes, as we increased the pressure on the lateral knee. This convinced us that the patient's pain was due in large measure to the piriformis syndrome in spite of other clinical considerations. We gave him a trigger point injection under EMG guidance, and he seemed to improve 20–30% immediately. Nevertheless, given the likelihood of the severe pain returning, we sent him for an emergency MRI.

An hour later we learned that he had a moderately large L5 herniation on the right side with a free fragment squeezing his L5 nerve root. When we called him, the pain was 6/10, and he readily accepted a phoned-in narcotic prescription and the names of two surgeons. The piriformis injection had helped him, but it was not directed to his principal problem after all. The psoriasis was irrelevant.

Acting on a Hunch

A 64-year-old consultant came in early June with a 4 weeks history of significant lower back pain without radiation. The pain vanished with therapy, but recurred in August whenever he bent forward for more than 3 or 4 min, e.g., washing dishes. X rays revealed mild retrolisthesis in the lumbar spine with well-preserved disc spaces.

Everything in the physical examination and EMG was normal except for a few positive sharp waves bilaterally at L5-S1. We asked him to lie in lateral decubitus and 65° of flexion at the hips for 5 min and repeated the H reflexes. There was no change from their normal values in the anatomical position.

We then asked him to stand and bend forward over the examination table on which he had previously been lying and we conducted serial H reflexes in this awkward position. In doing so, we were replicating the weight-bearing and gravitational effects of what actually caused the pain. After 4 min, he felt the pain. After 5 min, there was a 4.3 ms delay in the left posterior tibial H reflex.

We concluded that it was the narrowing of the canal by the action of gravity on his retrolisthesis that probably caused the radiculopathy and was definitely responsible for his pain, rather than any simple structural neuroforaminal encroachment. We successfully treated him with abdominal and extensor strengthening, Alexander technique postural work, and gave him an abdominal binder.

Right to Bare Arms

A 44-year-old ex-military man working as a physical trainer in a health club complained of left medial forearm tingling, predominantly when raising his arm in abduction with straightened elbow. He cited a history of a deep gash in his left upper arm and was considering surgery for what he believed to be adhesions restraining/entrapping his ulnar nerve when he abducted. We tested bilateral conductions from Erb's point to the first dorsal interosseous muscle (needle electrode) bilaterally at rest, with nearly identical NCV and F waves, and small variation in CMAP's. EMG was normal. Placing the arm and re-testing the ulnar nerve in extreme abduction, and then in the extremes of flexion, extension and adduction, Adson's maneuver and internal rotation with extension did nothing to change any of these metrics. Sensory NCVs were borderline low, and SNAPs were somewhat small for bilateral median, ulnar, and radial nerves.

We advised him to skip the surgery, and he did. One year later, he was diagnosed with a peripheral neuropathy of the diabetic type. At that time, his hemoglobin A1C was 6.1.

Ironing with a Wrinkle

A 5-year resident of the United States from Italy presented in February with no immediate complaint, telling us we had to do something, his right arm was allergic to Spring. Every year since coming here, he related, his arm began to hurt by mid-May, and became nearly intolerable in early June, only to resolve by the 4th of July. Conventional physical examination and EMG were normal. "What do you expect?" he exclaimed, "It isn't even March yet." We re-tested his median NCV across the pronator teres, this time in extreme active pronation. There was a delay of 1.1 ms on the right, but also a delay of 0.8 ms for similar conductions on the left.

We inquired into his activities. It turned out that in his community, brides wore elaborate crinolines and other garments that required heroic amounts of ironing. And in that community, he was the man. We advised him to go shopping and secure an iron with a handle that limited pronation. He brought us a few examples that fit the bill. The problem never reappeared, although at last contact business was still relatively brisk and seasonal.

Taking Matters to Extremes

A 37-year-old right-handed man who often used a shovel presented with left posterolateral upper arm pain that worsened as his work day went on. He had had many knocks and minor accidents in his life, but nothing distinctly connected with the onset of the pain 4 months ago nor its intensifying over the past 6 weeks. He had already had a normal MRI of the cervical spine and a normal standard EMG of both upper extremities and paraspinal musculature.

Physical examination was essentially normal, with no sensory changes. Provocative testing revealed a strongly positive (and painful) Adson's maneuver on the affected left side, but not on the right. Since his complaints were purely sensory, we studied radial SSEP to Erb's point and the somatosensory strip in the anatomical position, which was normal on the right side and mildly prolonged on the left. We tried to compare these values with what would be seen in Adson's maneuver, but it was too painful for the patient to hold the position long enough to acquire even 10 evoked responses.

We tried conductions from Erb's point to the extensor indicis proprius and the teres minor. Both were normal in the anatomical position; both were significantly prolonged, from 4.8 to 5.8 and from 2.4 to 4.8, respectively, in Adson's maneuver. We had the normal cervical MRI and EMG: the cervical spine was decidedly not involved. But the question still remained: where was the injury? We still had too many diagnoses: the problem could be in the posterior divisions, in the cords, the radial nerve, or its branches.

The patient was considering surgery in the apical region; the pain was severe, and he figured that soon he would be disabled. We felt that might be the wrong decision and might actually lead to greater pain and disability; so we took an extreme measure: we repeated the stimulations at Erb's point under extreme or exaggerated Adson's maneuver. Conductions to the extensor indicis proprius were unchanged, but the proximal motor latency to the teres minor was increased to a whopping 6.9 ms.

Over the next 4 weeks, using myofascial release, manual medical techniques and postural changes, and insisting that the patient wear a figure-of-eight brace, we worked successfully to free the axillary nerve from unseen and never discovered problems at or near the thoracic outlet. The patient's problem essentially disappeared, though he also began at times to shovel "left-handed." We did not have the opportunity to test him again, but the way things broke down is shown in Table 10.1.

Table 10.1 Extreme conditions brought out the likely pathogenetic mechanism, the likely pain generator here

Anatomic	Adson's	Extreme Adson's	Supination
EIP = 4.8	5.8	5.8	5.9
Contralateral	4.8	4.8	4.9
T. minor = 2.4	4.8	**6.9**	

The extreme response to the extreme version of Adson's maneuver here revealed that the pathology was in the fibers of the axillary nerve.

It's Not All in the Wrist!

A 41-year-old right-handed small and slender guitar-playing song-writer presented with right palmar cramping after playing for 20–30 min. Conventional EMG with NCV and MRI of the cervical spine and upper extremities were essentially normal. We asked her to bring in her guitar. She after two songs in which she strummed with a plectrum, the cramping arose. The back and forth motion of her wrist prompted us to check her ulnar conductions below the elbow, where the nerve runs between fibers of the lateral head of the flexor carpi ulnaris. After obtaining a baseline, we asked her to go into extreme medial (ulnar) deviation while holding the plectrum, and repeated the conductions to the first dorsal interosseous muscle. There was a delay of 1.4 ms, nearly 45% of the total conduction time. We repeated the same comparison on the left (without the two songs) finding no discrepancy between values seen in the anatomical and the medially deviated position. We asked her to return to her best guitar teacher, and wrote her a note to tell her the problem. The problem slowly resolved over the next 4 months: The patient had to hold the guitar slightly lower, move her arm a little more, and the wrist a little less.

Driving for a Stretch

A 44-year-old financial executive had pain in her right buttock when driving her little car. She had a very slight sensory deficit at the right dorsal lateral foot, but otherwise a normal physical examination, and normal MRI and standard EMG. We replicated the conditions of driving her low-slung car, a naturally occurring provocative test, with no success. We then compared her H reflexes in the anatomical position with those seen when one-by-one the hips were flexed to 90°, that knee totally extended, and the ipsilateral foot in extreme dorsiflexion. The left H reflex did not change, but the right was delayed by 1.0 ms. In a confirmatory sign, the patient volunteered that she felt buttock pain after the right leg was held the position for 10–20 s, but not the left.

We believe it was important to retain the contralateral hip and knee in 180° of extension, i.e., the conventional straight-leg-raise test position, in order to retain the pelvis in neutral or mildly forward-tilted position. Otherwise we would not have stretched the fibers of the sciatic nerve itself.

We worked with myofascial release near the linea aspera to free fibers of the peroneal nerve especially, since the numbness was at the dorsal and dorsolateral foot. The patient improved very quickly in this case and made a fairly long (and painless) motor trip a month later.

Exclusive Considerations

A 45-year-old healthcare accountant presented with increased left-sided sciatic pain and numbness of the sole of the foot and distal calf that were exacerbated by straight-leg raise. She had had a normal MRI 1 year before, when the sensory deficit but not the pain appeared, and a normal EMG apart from delay of the left H reflex with flexion, adduction, and internal rotation (FAIR test). Sensation returned to normal after successful treatment for piriformis syndrome then.

In the current examination, there was buttock tenderness, but the FAIR test was normal. This time the 3-min extension test was negative. Because of these negative results, where what were once diagnoses of exclusion had been excluded, we looked beyond the lumbar spine deep down in the sacrum. There were impressive positive sharp waves at S3 and in the peroneus longus.

Repeat MRI showed a midline disc herniation at L4-5, which apparently was only affecting the rootlets that became the S3 nerve root as they passed by L4-5 in the lumbar spine. We treated her with McKenzie-type exercises. She was slow to improve at first, but after 8 weeks was 60–75% better.

A Turn for the Worse

A 34-year-old policeman came to us fully worked up and partially treated 5 months after a patrol car accident had caused moderate bilateral disc herniations at C5-C6-C7 and T1 that were detected on MRI. EMG revealed bilateral denervation at all those levels; physical therapy had helped 8/10 pain decrease to 2–3/10. The problem was that when he turned his head to the left, either looking in side-view mirrors or entering/exiting the car, he felt pain and paraesthesias along the medial aspect of his left arm to his little finger. He said it made him miserable every time. It was reliable, he could count on it. He was not seeking disability, but he could no longer work in a squad car. He wanted a desk job.

Rather than repeat the entire EMG, we focused on F waves of bilateral median and ulnar nerves in the anatomical position vs. with left lateral rotation. The left median F wave averaged 26.7 ms in the anatomical position; the left ulnar F wave varied between 33.0 and 34.0 ms in the anatomical position, averaging 33.2 ms. He had to remain left laterally rotated for close to half a minute before he felt the paraesthesias, and before we saw the F waves vary beyond their previous limits. After 1 min, the left median F waves averaged 27.8–28.2 ms; left ulnar F wave was prolonged to 35.6 ms - 2.4 ms beyond its average in the anatomical position. At that point the paraesthesias were bearable but severe.

We reported these changes to the police surgeon, and the patient was given a desk job.

Having seen a number of examples of "plinthside creativity" that resolved ambiguous situations, some readers may feel that there are other instances in which provocative and evocative maneuvers might be studied, and helpful rules of thumb, guidelines, or actual parameters developed. In the final part of the final chapter, we shall attempt to aid any such efforts with our experience, such as it is, hoping to help investigators sidestep some of the difficulties that we have encountered. We approach this in a question-and-answer format.

Who If Not We?

Anyone attempting to find useful ways of combining the physical examination with EMG, using electrophysiological means to quantify the pathological effects of functional and positional changes, many of which are brought out by physical examination, will likely think of most of the considerations we are about to mention. Still, if it functions as nothing more than a check-list, what follows may have some value to the inquiring electromyographer. There is a wealth of physical examination lore, much of considerable clinical import, and much of which may be overlooked in the races for sharper MRIs, better surgical techniques, and genetic understanding of disease.

While these high-tech endeavors deserve at least the energetic dedication they currently enjoy, the physical examination remains an innocuous and economical means of securing diagnoses and directing and at times bypassing the more highly technical aspects of contemporary medical care. But the physical examination has been neglected in teaching and in practice. Who are better fit than we, physiatrists and neurologists, to develop a fusion of electrodiagnosis and the physical examination to the betterment of our craft and science, and the understanding of our patients' problems?

- *Muscular and Bony Anatomy*
  It is one thing to know the brachial and lumbosacral plexes, and another to understand their environment: the movement patterns and dynamic interactions of the muscles, connective tissue, and bones that surround neural tissues, govern their movements in the body, and either protect or entrap them. We have found that the anatomical variations that exist, e.g., in cervical ribs, arterial and venous elements encircling nerves, congenitally narrow spinal canals, and piriformis muscle–sciatic nerve perforations, are far less commonly pathogenetic than normal kinesiological relationships stretched to their limits, habitually overused or abused.

  But if anyone is equipped to study action patterns—from gross balance to girls' basketball, muscle synergies—from multiple sclerosis to the concert piano, coordination—from movement disorders to health club ergonomics, it is the people who do EMG. It would be hard to find another group of clinical electrophysiologists that might transition so easily from the staid and static, nearly uniform technique of current EMG practice to a dynamic investigation of many true-to-life neuromuscular problems.
- *Kinesiology*
  Knowing the moving parts is important; learning how they move relative to one another is a lifetime business. Consider the mathematics professor who refused to turn his back completely to his students. From time to time he would have a sharp pain in his shoulder and even drop the chalk with which he was writing. Before he had surgery for a mild acromioclavicular impingement seen on X rays, we realized that this activity approximated the Allen test, and after the maneuver produced significant median F-wave prolongation in NCV testing, we found that a 10–20° shift in his stance eliminated his problem.

  A middle-aged right-handed poet was having episodes of posterior shoulder pain and simultaneous changes in her handwriting. Many diagnoses were entertained until, on the Internet one night she learned that the infraspinatus draws the hand across the page it is writing. Ultrasound found no calcific tendonitis, so she came to a physiatrist. A mild impingement at the thoracic outlet was worsened by the slumping posture she assumed in provocative conductions from Erbs point.

The cure was apparent when she said "But that's exactly the way I sit when I'm really working."

One intriguing area in kinesiology is the shoulder. The scapula is nearly uniquely unfixed to its bony attachments. Only the terminal digits and the hyoid bone have similar freedom. The scapula wanders far (but not aimlessly) over the posterior thorax: the kinesiology of its coordinated muscles, the strength, and timing of their concentric and eccentric contractions are the heart and soul of useful rehabilitation and effective orthopedic surgery.

The other region in which kinesiology is king is the pelvis: here the movement of the constituent bones is actually quite minimal, since so many of them are fused. But this is true for the same reason that the pelvis is so fascinating: it is built, particularly in the upright human, for support. If the free-wheeling scapula favors flexibility and versatility, the closely knit sacrum, the flying buttress hips and the Roman arch they make together with the sacrum as keystone, favor support.

What this means, of course, is that the muscles work in reverse in the pelvis: In walking, the gluteus medius contracts not to abduct the leg, but to keep the contralateral pelvis from sinking during swing phase. Eccentric anterior tibialis contractions keep us from slapping the floor with each forward step. This shift in the function of muscles may explain some of physiologists' fascination with the pelvis. It certainly explains why muscles of the pelvis, with their constant supporting roles, may cause prolonged aches and nerve damage difficult to associate with any particular movement. This knowledge of the shoulder and pelvic girdles has enabled the studies in this book and many others

- *Peripheral Neurology*

  If there is anything that distinguishes physiatrists and EMG-adept neurologists from our fellows, it is knowledge of the peripheral nervous system and beneficial use of that knowledge. It is, of course, a *sine qua non* in using provocative and evocative maneuvers to extend the scope of the physical examination with electrodiagnosis.

  Obviously anyone extending the scope of EMG must do EMG, and that is the point here. A radiologist may wait for advances in physics, infectious disease gets its boosts from genetics and pharmacology, and orthopedic surgeons welcome new alloys and prosthetic designs. But if there is no advance in electrophysiology, to mildly mutilate a famous phrase, "the fault, dear colleague is not in our suppliers but in ourselves."

- *EMG*

  In some quarters the electrophysiological examination is as perfunctory as drawing blood: little is communicated about the patient's history, and apart from standard measures and probings, little is done. This approach is unlikely to lead to discovering a functional diagnosis. To do the type of thing advocated in this book, the examining physician is obliged truly to examine the patient and be aware of a fairly extensive review of systems as relates to the chief complaint(s).

  Just mentally thumbing through some of the clinical sketches presented above may provide a sharp contrast to the immaculate case presentations in some of

Medicine's leading journals. Assessing the moving parts, which leads to so many functional diagnoses, requires some familiarity with *what* the patient does, and *when* pathological things occur are the first steps to determining how and why.

- *Functional Approach to Patient*

  We physicians are frequently labeled materialists because of our reliance on concrete entities for pathogenesis: a broken bone, a space-occupying mass, a foramen of one kind or another that is no longer patent. But looking at the relationship between moving parts is as abstract as differential calculus, and this relationship is an increasingly common source of pain and disability (and eventually material injury) in the ever more technological world in which we are less and less doing what comes naturally.

  How much do you have to know? How familiar should one be with the Reformer to judge whether Pilates is causing the problem? Which genetic combinations lead to myelin disorders that favor episodic entrapment? One thing is sure: in this situation, more is more: the eye sees what the mind knows, and another candidate for cliche: if you do not seek, you will not find.

- *Treatment*

  Those that diagnose a condition generally treat it. Functional pathology is no exception. Physical and occupational therapists and the numerous injection and bracing techniques are generally close at hand to the electromyographer. It is often non-trivial to devise effective treatment for functional pathology, even though it eventually turns out to be quite simple in a number of cases.

  Being able to use the same maneuver on serial occasions to assess the efficacy of given treatments is a boon to physical and occupational therapists. Being able to do serial electrodiagnostic testing validates the method of diagnosis, and also confirms the utility of treatment. This is what we did with botulinum neurotoxins A and B and physical therapy in Chapters 5 and 7. We did essentially the reverse, using therapeutic success to support the utility of H reflexes in extension in Chapter 8.

Surgery

Somatosensory evoked potentials (SSEP) during scoliosis surgery might be considered an early instance of "provocative electrodiagnostic technique." In the Harrington rod procedure, for example, stimuli are initiated at the ankle, with pick-ups at the somatosensory strip, well above the surgical area. Latencies are tested before the laminar hooks are tightened into place and directly afterwards. If the potentials change very much at all, either in interpeak latencies or amplitude, the hooks are immediately loosened. Here the functional change is provided by the surgeon's tightening (and possibly subsequently loosening) a sort of winch that changes the conformation of the spine.

There may be other uses for intraoperative functional electrophysiological testing, involving surgeries for the three conditions we have written about here, as well

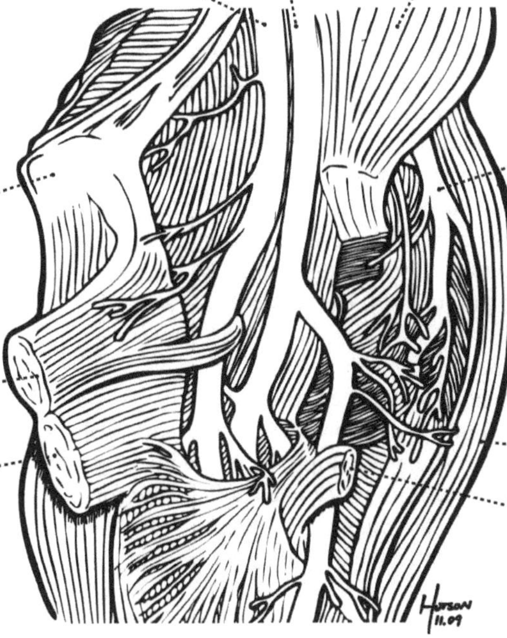

Fig. 10.4 Pronating against resistance may tighten the slip of muscular tissue that surrounds the median nerve, as we saw with the man seasonally ironing crinolines

as others. An example might be surgery for pronator entrapment of the median nerve, in which an intraoperative conduction across that level in (passive) pronation vs. supination might be a safer way to a positive outcome. The same conductions performed pre-operatively both in (active) flexion and extension might be helpful in determining the likely success of the procedure (Fig. 10.4).

The Tools of the Trade

This is not a high-tech endeavor, at least not yet. In provocative maneuvers, there is often a certain amount of pressure exerted in one way or another. Some control over it is obviously desirable. One or two strain gauges are helpful to regulate how much force is exerted with some degree of uniformity, e.g., in Adson's maneuver or in flexion, adduction, and internal rotation.

The correlation between the independent variable, how extreme the provocative maneuver is, and the dependent variable, how much change it brings about in the electrophysiological parameter, is something that can be observed even without the gauges, but refining the technique beyond what we present here would be desirable.

In an earlier paper [1], we inverted a strain gauge and applied its handle to the superficial branch of the radial sensory nerve as it crossed the radial styloid, in an effort to demonstrate that temporary pressure can reversibly decrease nerve conduction velocity in humans. We found that less than 5 pounds of force reversibly delayed radial conductions by a full millisecond. Hong et al. have shown this quite conclusively in animal studies [2].

The only other ubiquitously useful tool is a statistical manner of relating the provocative or evocative maneuver with electrophysiological change. In simple cases, *t* tests may be sufficient, but in the complex situations one may find in the operating room or the cancer ward, far more sophisticated analysis might be required to show the correlation. The essential thing is to define the ranges in which one expects the relationship to hold. But then what?

- *Establish Normals*
  This is where the pressure gauges come in handy: to establish that under the same amount of strain, there is a different response—probably no response—in people who do not have the signs or symptoms under investigation. It is useful to have a few "positive" cases first in order to establish how much pressure you will need to equal what evokes the changes in people with the condition under scrutiny, when you test those that ostensibly do not have it.
- *Standard Deviations*
  Standard deviations, introduced so long ago by Christian Gauss, are still the stock in trade of statistical significance. Calculating the standard deviation of the parametric changes seen in normals during the provocative or evocative maneuver is critical for establishing a benchmark value above which one identifies the condition. The idea, of course, is to estimate how likely or better how unlikely it is to come upon the given value "by chance."
- *Statistical Significance vs. Clinical Significance*
  The industry standard for this is 2 standard deviations beyond the mean. In a normal population, that yields a $p < 0.05$. We have generally chosen to identify patients with values greater than 3 standard deviations beyond the mean seen in normals. We use the standard deviation of the change seen with the provocative maneuver in the piriformis test. However the H reflexes we studied pass the point of functional compression (the piriformis muscle) twice: both in the afferent and efferent limbs of the reflex; so 3 standard deviations seemed reasonable. Other metrics may have clinical utility, i.e., denote treatable conditions, in other cases, but avoiding of false positives will always be a statistical matter.

  At first, one always has what seems to be perforce an arbitrary determination of what is significant. One tries to determine what level of deviation from normal indicates a treatable diagnosis, a pathological condition causing the patient's symptoms. But the 2 or 3 SD (0.05 or 0.005) mark may be a good starting place, a way to select patients, and a basis from which to make finer delineations later.

  One example was the question of whether changes in position could develop clinically relevant spinal stenosis in patients with spondylolisthesis. This meant testing people without spondylolisthesis and eventually analyzing them in terms of what we found. But at first, we had to isolate a real and replicable electrophysiological effect of extension.

- *What Does It Mean?*
  Many findings are useful although they are non-specific. A "spot on the lung" may be tuberculosis, a bleb, or much worse; finding it does not determine the diagnosis, rather it determines the clinician to find the cause. Studies of sensitivity and specificity help here, and are the obverse of a diagnosis of exclusion: they allow one to make clinical decisions in the context of several conditions.

  This is where provocative and evocative tests are at their best. If Gaenslen's sign reproduces the patient's symptoms, then the lower back pain is plausibly linked to sacroiliac joint derangement. For example, if Gaenslen's sign is present and there are paraesthesias, then the diagnostic work is not finished. But if the paraesthesias are in a dermatomal distribution, then they are more specific than Gaenslen's sign and are trump.
- *Making It Useful: Treat Patients Identified by the Tests, Based on the Pathology*
  This is so obvious it is almost embarrassing to state. Obvious, but not always easy. After finding a test for piriformis syndrome, we were not sure how to treat it. Fortunately we received a generous outpouring of methods, techniques, and cautions from the worldwide therapeutic community. What we have just about always experienced is that when you "discover" a new technique for a clinical entity that seemed so murky, there are a surprising number of other clinicians who have found it before and discovered or invented adroit and effective means to treat it! The Internet is a fantasy-like advantage here.
- *Follow Results with the Functional Test*
  One happy aspect of functional pathology is that very commonly it is reversible. Therefore, one can judge the efficacy of a treatment by repeating the functional test at appropriate intervals. If one finds that the clinical signs and symptoms vary directly with the abnormality of the electrophysiological test, it is not that unlikely that the test reflects the underlying pathology.

  This goes for pre-and post-surgical conditions as well. See Drs. Ringel and Webber's work on page 22 of Chapter 7.

  But the clinical course does not always mirror effective treatment very closely. People often convalesce for months after antibiotics are stopped and the pneumonia is cured. In nerve injuries due to functional conditions, the same may be true. Myelin sheaths and injured axons may take some time to return, or may never return to baseline. In other words, removing the cause is one thing, but the effect may linger on. Being present at a few surgeries, if that is part of the treatment of the condition, can help determine whether the vaso nervorum or the substance of the nerve sheaths have been denuded or affected at all.
- *Improve Treatment and Surgery*
  When there is a technique that helps the condition, functional EMG gives ways of evaluating how much it helps, and after how many treatments. Functional EMG may also furnish an objective method to decide between physical therapeutic and surgical techniques, through post-treatment testing. In longer-term practice it might help decide which treatment is best for which circumstances.

This Book As a Provocative/Evocative Maneuver

We hope that some readers will be interested in this aspect of EMG, and that the many flaws in this book will not turn them away, but rather stimulate them to do better.

References

1. Fishman, LM, Zybert, PA. "Electrophysiological evidence of piriformis syndrome." *Arch Phys Med Rehabil.* 1992 Apr;73(4):359–64.
2. Hong, C-Z. "Reversible conduction block in polyneuropathy after ultrasound at therapeutic dosage." *Arch Phys Med Rehabil.* 1988;69:746.

Index

Note: The letters 'f' and 't' following locators refer to figures and tables respectively.

L.M. Fishman, A.N. Wilkins, *Functional Electromyography*,
DOI 10.1007/978-1-60761-020-5,

F

MIX
Papier aus verantwortungsvollen Quellen
Paper from responsible sources
FSC® C105338
FSC
www.fsc.org

If you have any concerns about our products,
you can contact us on
ProductSafety@springernature.com

In case Publisher is established outside the EU,
the EU authorized representative is:
Springer Nature Customer Service Center GmbH
Europaplatz 3, 69115 Heidelberg, Germany

Printed by Libri Plureos GmbH
in Hamburg, Germany